Contents

Contributors

Lynne Allan is the Coordinator of Student Field Education in a large government human service organisation in Victoria, Australia. Lynne is a social worker who has worked in the youth field and extensively in the area of domestic violence. She has held various teaching roles, in the university and vocational education and training (VET) sectors. Lynne began working and studying in this field in 1990, completing qualifications in welfare, social work and family therapy, and a Master's in Professional Practice Development. Lynne has a passionate interest in the education of students and their practice, and how critical reflection can contribute to this.

Janet Allen is a registered social worker and lecturer in Dalhousie University's School of Social Work. Prior to her work in social work education, Janet worked as a health policy researcher in the field of women's health and as a clinical social worker with women survivors of sexual trauma. Her varied research interests and experience include spirituality and clinical social work practice, critically reflective methodologies, diversity and organisational change, and social work pedagogy.

Gurid Aga Askeland is Associate Professor in social work at Diakonhjemmet University College. She developed and implemented the distance education programme in social work in Norway. She has been a guest lecturer in master's programmes in social work throughout Norway, and also Ethiopia and Italy. She was Chair of the Nordic Committee of Schools of Social Work for four years, and has also been a member of the Board of International Association of Schools of Social Work for 10 years. She is on the editorial boards of the *European Journal of Social Work* and *International Social Work*. Her books include (with Malcolm Payne) *Globalization and International Social Work: Postmodern Change and Challenge* (Aldershot: Ashgate, 2008). She has edited a book and published and co-authored some articles on critical reflection.

Gail Baikie is an Assistant Professor at the School of Social Work, Dalhousie University. She has had a lengthy professional career primarily related to the social development of Indigenous peoples. This interest carries over into her teaching and research. In particular, she has embraced and evolved the Fook/Gardner critical reflection model into a method for decolonising and decolonialising the minds of professionals and researchers. The identification and development of decolonising and indigenous methods for research, professional development and social work practice is an extension of this interest.

Jeffrey Gordon Baker is a social worker and an artist. Originally from the United States, he currently lives and works in London. He has worked in the fields of mental health, corrections, early childhood education and statutory children's services, and as a practice educator for student social workers. He has an undergraduate degree from New York University, a Master of Social Work degree from Hunter College School of Social Work/City University of New York, and an MA from Central St Martins/University of the Arts London. In 2012 he will begin work on a PhD in the department of Psychosocial Studies at Birkbeck College, University of London.

Jodi Butler is a Master of Social Work graduate from the Dalhousie School of Social Work. Jodi's research framework is grounded in feminist principles and her research interests include the construction of helper/client identity binaries, health/illness discourse in professional and peer communities, and the gender analysis of mental health policy and practice. Her past research has included collaborative work exploring the experiences of women involved in the justice system and an auto-ethnographic study of 'illness' identity. She is currently involved in a research project investigating the online Critical Reflection Dialogue Group.

Carolyn Campbell is an Assistant Professor at the School of Social Work, Dalhousie University. As an educator and social worker she has focused on congruency between the content and processes of education for critical practice, especially related to concepts of difference, privilege and social justice. She is passionate about social work education and has participated in extensive curricular design and development, taught a wide range of courses, offered numerous workshops, and been honoured to participate in students' processes of transformational learning.

Clare Delany is a senior lecturer and Director of Teaching and Learning at the School of Health Sciences, The University of Melbourne and a Senior Ethics Associate at the Children's Bioethics Centre at the Royal Children's Hospital in Melbourne. Clare has Master's degrees in Health and Medical Law and Physiotherapy (manipulation). Her PhD and ongoing research interests include legal and ethical obligations of health practitioners; the role of critical reflection in clinical education; healthcare communication; and ways of implementing ethical theory into clinical practice.

Yolande Ferguson completed a four-year social work degree at the University of Stellenbosch in South Africa and has worked in the UK as a social worker for the past eight years in several different social work teams. She currently works in professional development of social work. Yolande facilitates critical reflection with newly qualified social workers and a staff group of supervisors from a residential unit. She has also been a practice assessor of student social workers since 2006.

Jan Fook travels internationally to conduct training in critical reflection. She has published widely in the area. In 2002 she established the Centre for Professional Development at La Trobe University, Australia, which specialises in short-course critical reflection training. She is currently Professor and Director of the School of Social Work at Dalhousie University, Canada, and also holds visiting appointments at Royal Holloway, University of London; St George's, University of London; and Kingston University (London). She is involved in organising an Economic and Social Research Council (UK)-funded seminar series entitled 'Critical Reflection: The Research Way Forward'. She is an Academician of the Academy of Social Sciences (UK).

Fiona Gardner has worked in social work for over 30 years in direct practice, management, teaching and research. In 1996, she established the Social Work Program at the LaTrobe Rural Health School, La Trobe University in Bendigo, where she is currently Head of Department. She also continues to run Centre for Professional Development workshops, primarily on critical reflection, supervision and spirituality. Her recent research includes training in spirituality/pastoral care and palliative care, and exploring a community-based approach to issues related to death and dying, including spirituality. She has co-authored two books on critical reflection and recently published a book on critical spirituality.

Roslyn Giles is an honorary senior lecturer in social work and policy studies, University of Sydney and recently retired from the position of Director of Social Work Field Education. This role brought together her extensive experience as a social work practitioner and manager, as a field education supervisor, and as a tertiary social work educator. Roslyn is very interested in the processes of adult learning, particularly combining life experiences with formal processes of critical reflection in striving for just and ethical practice. Her research includes projects to develop and implement national social work practice standards, as well as health context practice-based data-mining projects and research about social work priorities in practice.

Belinda Hearne has a professional background which includes qualifications in psychiatric nursing and social work, and she completed a Master's of Professional Practice Development from La Trobe University in 2006. She has practised counselling and nursing and worked as a manager in a range of sectors, including child and family, drug and alcohol, and mental health. Belinda is currently the Director of a program delivering services to current and ex-serving veterans and family members who have served or currently serve in the Australian Defence Force.

Helen Hickson is a social worker and lecturer at La Trobe University in Australia. She was inspired by a half-day critical reflection workshop run by the Centre for Development at La Trobe University, and is currently enrolled in a PhD there, exploring the ways in which social workers learn, teach and use critical reflection in their professional practice.

Sinéad McGilloway is Senior Lecturer and Director of the Mental Health and Social Research Unit (MHSRU), Department of Psychology, National University of Ireland, Maynooth. She is a community and public health psychologist with 20 years' experience in undertaking applied, policy-relevant health and social care research. Dr McGilloway has researched, secured grants and published widely on a broad range of health and social care topics including, in particular, child and adult mental health and service evaluation. She has authored and co-authored numerous publications, including peer-reviewed papers; books/volumes; book chapters; commissioned research reports; conference proceedings, papers and abstracts; and articles of professional interest.

Kathleen McLoughlin is Head of Education, Research and Professional Development at Milford Care Centre, a specialist palliative care service based in Limerick, Ireland. She graduated with a first-class honours degree in psychology from the University of Luton in 1995, and is currently completing a doctorate in psychology at the National University of Ireland, Maynooth under the supervision of Dr Sinéad McGilloway. Kathleen has adapted the Fook and Gardner (2007) model to inform the development of a short course for health professionals working with death, dying and palliative care.

Christine Morley BSW (Hons) PhD is Associate Professor of Social Work in the School of Social Sciences, Faculty of Arts and Business at the University of the Sunshine Coast, Queensland, Australia. Formerly at Deakin University in Victoria, she has been teaching, practising and researching critical reflection over the past 14 years. She completed her PhD using critical reflection as a methodology, and she has published widely using critical reflection as her inspiration.

Rosalie Pockett is a senior lecturer in Social Work & Policy Studies at the University of Sydney. She has a career background in hospital/health social work practice, and her areas of research interest include health inequalities; interprofessional education and practice; leadership and management in social work; professional practice supervision; and the transition of new graduates to the workplace. A particular focus of these research interests is in practice-based research inquiry. Her recent work in critical reflection includes its use in social work student education and as a theoretical framework for practice research.

Riki Savaya is Head of the Bob Shapell School of Social Work at Tel Aviv University, Israel. Her research, which employs both quantitative and qualitative methods, focuses on various aspects of professional practice.

These aspects encompass the uses, outcomes and impacts of information technology in social service agencies; evaluation of social programmes; features and challenges of practice with minority groups and populations at risk; and social workers' daily practices and experiences as revealed in their critical reflections. She has published over 60 papers in peer-reviewed journals and about the same number of research and evaluation reports. Her work is underpinned by the endeavour to gain scientific knowledge to improve social work practice.

Eddie Taalman has worked for 32 years as an occupational therapist in the medical arena. His early career was spent in eastern rural Victoria, acute regional services. In Melbourne, he has spent the past 27 years in sub-acute rehabilitation. In that time, additional studies in health services management have led to a passion for team dynamics and team-building. In 2007 he was part of a Southern Health working party to develop supervision guidelines, and was appointed project officer to coordinate and implement a supervision package across sub-acute and ambulatory care services. He currently is employed as the Manager of Occupational Therapy, Dandenong, Victoria

Gavan Thomson grew up in the Riverina area of New South Wales, Australia, which left him with an interest in rural issues. He completed an applied science degree, then worked in hospital labs as a research technician. This led to interest in social health and political change. He undertook a graduate diploma in community health. From there he become a communard at Commonground, and pursued counselling by undertaking a graduate diploma in loss and grief counselling. He then studied social work at La Trobe University, Bendigo. For the past nine years he has been the Coordinator of a School Focused Youth Service at Cobaw Community Health, a developmental program which builds a better system to support at-risk young people.

Jackie Thornhill is a graduate of the Bachelor of Social Work program at Dalhousie University and a practising social worker in a progressive mental health setting. Since 2007, Jackie has been involved in the facilitation of critical reflection discussions and has investigated the use of dialogue groups and critical reflection in educational settings. Jackie's theoretical framework is informed largely by critical theory and feminism. She has an interest in research and practice related to gender, sexuality and women's experiences with sexual violence.

Deborah Watkin is a physiotherapist working in public health in Melbourne, Australia, who has completed a Master's of Professional Practice Development in critical reflection, and acted as facilitator for the initial study described in her chapter. She has also completed a research project in a clinical setting in relation to clinical educator perspectives on factors affecting student learning in clinical placements.

1 Critical reflection in context
Contemporary perspectives and issues

Jan Fook

Why this book?

The idea that some form of reflection is seen as a necessary ingredient of professional practice is quite familiar (Polkinghorne, 2004). This idea is supported in a range of professions and disciplines (Fook et al., 2006). Yet there are several aspects to this which still remain relatively unclear and are therefore problematic for any attempts to introduce, and sustain, reflection in particular settings.

Foremost amongst these problems is the question of exactly what form the reflection takes. What approach and theoretical underpinning to reflection is being applied, and exactly how, in concrete terms, is this being practised? How does a worker or student demonstrate that they are reflective? Is reflection the same as reflective practice, and how does being 'critical' fit with these ideas? Is critical reflection the same as reflective practice or critical thinking, and does it matter?

The second problem is the challenge of changing contexts. Whilst there are undoubtedly more calls for critical reflection (Munro, 2011), economic constraints in many countries mean that workplace environments are more risk aversive and therefore often less willing to support workers to engage in reflective activities which might potentially undermine organisational goals. In addition, workplace 'tick-box' cultures can work against developing more amorphous reflective cultures, and simply finding the time to reflect becomes problematic with increased workloads.

Lastly, whilst critical reflection has been well developed for individual learning, especially in educational settings, much less is known about how it can be managed and sustained in particular organisational settings (Boud et al., 2006). What practical, ethical and organisational issues are involved in introducing and sustaining the practice and culture of critical reflection in particular contexts? In short, how do we 'organise' reflection? (Reynolds and Vince, 2004).

For some years, my colleague Fiona Gardner and I have worked with introducing, developing and teaching a particular model of critical reflection which is primarily group-based and can be modified for use in various settings. Different individuals and groups around the world have worked with us and have subsequently implemented this model in varying ways. We hope to make a contribution to addressing the problems outlined above through presenting their experiences and perspectives.

This book has three main aims:

- to showcase concrete ways of working with this critical reflection model in different settings, in order to contribute to continued improvement and application of the model;
- to illustrate concrete examples of the model's application, to assist professionals to apply it within their own context/organisation;
- to further conceptualise and develop the theory of critical reflection, through an explication of its practical application in a range of settings.

In this chapter I briefly review the major issues and challenges involved in how the practice of critical reflection needs to be developed. I also outline the particular model of critical reflection on which contributors have based their own practice of critical reflection, and provide an overview of the book's organisation and the content of the different chapters as they relate to our overall aims.

The increased need for critical reflection

What are the main current arguments about the needs for critical reflection? Clearly there have been longstanding appeals, going back to Socrates, about the need to reflect as part of the 'normal' requirements of a 'healthy' life (Polkinghorne, 2004), and these have never really receded. The current wonder, though, is that in times when the everyday work climate seems to run in the opposing direction, towards greater regulation, there are renewed calls for reflection to be incorporated into the everyday practice of individual professionals (Munro, 2011). There may be many good and bad reasons for this. Amongst the latter, it may be that reduced economic resources push the responsibility (and equivalent blame when it goes wrong) for quality practice onto individuals. On the upside, though, critical reflection is seen to be a way of addressing the need for organisations to learn (Hoyrup, 2004), increasing a sense of personal empowerment (Fook and Askeland, 2006), providing social and emotional support for workers (Ruch, 2007), and improving practice in a whole variety of ways (Fook and Gardner, 2007: 130–42). In addition, reflective approaches to practice may be seen as the appropriate way to conceptualise the kinds of judgement and complex practice that are needed from professionals (Polkinghorne, 2004). The need to address contextuality, and to find other ways of theorising practice and human experience that is less 'top-down' (Flyvberg, 2000), are all part of this greater call to make our understanding and practice more inclusive of different contexts and perspectives in changing circumstances. Critical reflection can play a key part in this greater context.

Current approaches and concepts relevant to critical reflection

Critical reflection (and related concepts of reflection, reflexivity and reflective practice) can be theorised in so many different ways. These terms are all used in a variety of disciplines, which do and do not cross-reference, so that the whole field can be vastly confusing. An overview of the literature indicates the following main theoretical frameworks, and indicates those that are under development.

Reflection

This is perhaps an older concept, and is related more to educational and philosophical literature. Major theorists include Dewey (1933), Kolb (1984) and Boud et al. (1985). These perspectives relate the idea of reflection to a process of learning from experience. Exactly how the learning takes place will depend on specific perspectives on learning, which may range from biological through psychodynamic, cognitive and psychological to more social perspectives, or combinations thereof such as socio-cultural (see Fenwick, 2000 for an outline of the major approaches). In essence, it involves the process of questioning the foundations of beliefs with a preparedness to change them in the light of that questioning. Of course, the concept of experience, and how it is theorised, also becomes important (Fook, 2011). The concept of reflection is also related to the idea of making meaning from experience, which in turn ties in with the uses of spirituality in critical reflection (see below).

Reflective practice

This perspective is exemplified most in the work of Donald Schön (1983), and relies heavily on the idea that tacit or implicit knowledge (or assumptions) are embedded in practice. Practice can therefore be improved by making such implicit knowledge explicit, thereby exposing it to scrutiny.

Reflexivity

This is a notion developed in the social sciences to refer to an acknowledgement of how our self plays a role in the knowledge that we recognise and develop: in short, how we see the world, others, and our place in relation to it and them. Being reflexive involves an ability to factor this knowledge into how professional decisions are made and acted upon. Taylor and White's (2000) work is a major example of how reflexivity can be applied in health and social care practice.

The linguistic turn

This concept refers to theories that focus on how our knowledge is made through the way we speak about it, and hence how we have a part in constructing our worlds and our 'reality'. Postmodern, poststructural and semiotic ways of thinking and researching are therefore relevant to critical reflection by providing an analysis of how power relations and arrangements may be supported unwittingly by the way we speak about our practice experience, in particular. The work of Foucault and the concept of discourse are integral to this analysis, as are the connections made between knowledge and power. Critical reflection, in this sense, can be likened to a process of deconstruction (and reconstruction) (Fook, 2012). The large body of work which uses narrative approaches to inform reflective practices is also relevant here (e.g. Taylor, 2006).

Critical perspectives

These perspectives include ways of theorising that make direct links between individual thinking and practice and the social and historical contexts in which they occur. This in turn provides an analysis of how power arrangements and relations might be maintained in individual practices. Awareness of these links can provide the basis for transformative change at individual levels. Brookfield (1995, 2005) is a major exponent of this type of critical approach to critical reflection.

Spirituality and Eastern religions

These perspectives are more recent contributions to the ways critical reflection is theorised and developed. The concept of spirituality introduces and develops the meaning aspect of critical reflection, which relates to the fundamentality of what is discovered and learnt about in the process (Hunt, 2010; Gardner, 2011). Such approaches emphasise the making of meaning based on a holistic connectedness and interconnectedness between individuals' experiences and the greater worlds in which they live. Other writers in this type of tradition refer to specific Buddhist concepts (Johns, 2005) or concepts such as the Tao (Humphrey, 2009).

Cognitive approaches

This type of approach is exemplified in the work of Mezirow and Associates (2000), whose approach to transformational learning includes critical reflection on assumptions. I categorise this approach as cognitive in that the emphasis is primarily on types and levels of thinking, with less emphasis on emotional aspects or broader social meanings.

Relational approaches

These approaches recognise the centrality of relationships and are seen as a reworking of earlier psychosocial and psychodynamic approaches (Ruch, 2009). Such approaches emphasise the need to address the emotional aspects of experience and the role of containing anxiety in this (Ruch, 2005). They may be seen as a contribution towards bridging the gap between the inner and outer worlds of individual experience.

Current issues

Organisational approaches

Organisational approaches emphasise the need for critical reflection to be incorporated into the organisational context in a way that contributes to learning, for the whole organisation, but which also benefits the needs of individual workers. Although there is a recognised need for individual reflection to contribute organisationally (Boud, 2010), it is not clear that both organisational and individual needs can be met mutually. This might be especially the case where it suits organisational cultures to blame individual practitioners. In other instances, it is by no means a foregone conclusion that organisations themselves can become reflective. Some authors prefer to speak of 'organising reflection' within an organisation (Reynolds and Vince, 2004) rather than of creating reflective organisations as a whole. The whole issue of how critical reflection can be practised and supported within specific organisational contexts is one that this book aims to address.

Practical understandings

A clear problem in developing critically reflective practices and environments is lack of clarity about what is understood by critical reflection and how it is played out in practice. In the fields of health and social care, there appears to be more literature on how reflection is taught in educational programmes (Fook et al., 2006) than on how it is actually practised within organisations (although there are some obvious exceptions, e.g. Gould and Baldwin, 2004). Even in teaching programs, the degree of detail about what is expected to be critically reflective, and the degree of detail about how it is to be assessed, can be variable and often vague (Norrie et al., 2012). For example, the rhetoric of critical reflection can be strong in broad course and program outlines, and less concrete in terms of learning content (literature and lecture material), assessment outlines and marking criteria. This book hopes to address this gap by pinning down some of the concrete detail involved in practising critical reflection.

Practical/ethical difficulties

Practical difficulties arise in exactly how critical reflection is incorporated into professional practice in a systematic and integrated way, especially with increased time and funding constraints. Should it be done in team meetings, as part of normal supervision activities (if they exist), or as part of a professional development program? Should critical reflection be mandatory? What are the ethical implications of individual workers divulging personal concerns or perceived mistakes in a monitoring environment? How can reflection best be aided in climates or cultures that are perceived to be judgemental or blaming? How much personal agency is really encouraged in cultures that appear to be controlling? And how does this learning, which primarily takes place for individual workers, become translated into organisational policy and practice and the culture of the workplace?

Outline of the model

The model built upon by contributors in this book has been developed over a period of time. Earlier versions were not published until 2000 (Napier and Fook, 2000) and 2002 (Fook, 2002), and the latter was an approach based more explicitly on concepts of deconstruction and reconstruction. Over the past 15 years, Fiona and I (separately and together) have conducted numerous training workshops based on this model, which was subsequently documented fully (Fook and Gardner, 2007). All of the contributors to this volume either have been trained by one of us at some stage, or have adopted a version of our model as a result of working with us or reading our material. Many of the contributors therefore worked with earlier versions of the model and have developed it further in their own ways. It is partly these modifications which we also wanted to document in this book, as they reflect to some extent the contexts for which the model was adapted.

In summary, the model is designed primarily for learning about professional practice, and is based upon a notion of critical reflection that involves the unsettling and examination of hidden assumptions in order to rework ideas and professional actions (Fook and Gardner, 2007: 21). The approach as documented in 2007 is underpinned by several theoretical/conceptual frameworks. These are: reflective practice; reflexivity; postmodernism; and critical perspectives. In summary, reflective practice draws upon the work of Donald Schön (1983) and emphasises the importance of tacit assumptions in influencing practice. The concept of reflexivity draws out the relevance of understanding how one's self can influence what and how knowledge is made, and can therefore shed light on how specific assumptions we make can arise from our own background and experience. Postmodern understandings point up the role of language and discourse in creating meanings and interpretations, and therefore knowledge and the exercise of power. Critical perspectives emphasise both how individual thinking/behaviours and social arrangements are linked, and therefore how individually held assumptions may emanate from a person's social environment. The latter is crucial in creating a vision for how social changes may be made by individuals, and therefore is an important ingredient in the potentially transformative aspect of critical reflection. Critical reflection, in this model, is about both unearthing hidden and powerful assumptions, and empowering individuals and creating a sense of agency. The model therefore does not sit solely within any of the perspectives as outlined above, but represents an amalgam of several approaches.

In later work, Fiona has developed the framework for critical reflection further by integrating it with an understanding of critical spirituality (see Gardner, 2011 and chapter 3 in this book). Essentially, critical spirituality refers to an overarching professional engagement with issues of spirituality and religion from a critical and holistic perspective. Such a perspective advocates practice that works with the whole person about what really matters to them in the context of their community, and from values of inclusion and social justice. In workshops, this has meant using the theories and processes of critical reflection in a more implicit form, so that participants in workshops engage in exercises that explore a range of experiences – past or current experiences, or those in the workshop itself that encourage articulating meaning at deeper levels.

In my own work, I have continued to develop what I term a more 'integrated' approach to critical reflection, which draws more on the 'learning from experience' aspect. I have therefore tended to speak more about critical reflection as overall being about learning from experience, simply initiated by unearthing hidden assumptions. This process is transformative in that it allows a fundamental reworking of experience (in an enabling way), which also functions as to provide new guidelines for action and an improvement of practice. In this way critical reflection can be applied to professional learning but also to the bigger task of living (Fook and Kellehear, 2010). This has meant that, when I now engage in critical reflection with groups of professionals, I tend to have a bigger project in mind when initiating the reflective process – not only is it about unearthing assumptions, but it is also about getting to the meaning, the crux or heart of the matter, including the emotional aspect (Fook, 2010) for whoever is reflecting. With this in mind, I have continued to work on developing the culture of critical reflection, being mindful of how to create climates that enable this bigger picture to develop (Fook, in press).

In practice, the original model relies on using discussion (usually in small groups) to assist individuals to reflect on a piece of their practice experience. The example of practice is normally a critical incident or a description of a concrete event on which the person chooses to reflect because it is significant to their learning in some way.

An appropriate learning climate is set up for the discussion. This climate is crucial to assisting reflection, as it is based on a learning culture that is not necessarily part of the mainstream or taken-for-granted approach to learning. It therefore must be made explicit and consciously maintained. It relies on principles of non-judgementality; of assisting with self-reflection rather than imposing views; of equality and inclusiveness in creating a space for different and contradictory views. Participants are guided to help with reflection by group members asking questions (e.g. 'what am I assuming about human relationships?'; 'what is coming out about my fundamental values?'; 'where does that thinking come from?'; 'how did my social context at the time have an influence?') informed by the different theoretical frameworks that underpin the approach. In this way, an understanding of different theories can aid reflection by providing different analyses of hidden assumptions and how they can be powerful. 'Power', and how it is understood, can have many meanings. What is emphasised is how particular understandings of power can illuminate the person's understanding of their own experience.

The discussion takes place in two structured stages: the first stage focuses on drawing out hidden assumptions, making minimal judgement of them. The emphasis in this first stage is being open to exposing assumptions in order to see where that leads. At the end of this first stage, each participant is asked to try to encapsulate what they think the main assumptions are that have come to light.

The second stage (usually conducted at a time separate from the first) focuses on the newer awarenesses that have emerged from the exposure of assumptions in the first stage. This stage is structured by drawing out the learning into broader guidelines, and making connections between the newer principles that emerge and how they might be practised. Participants are encouraged, at the end of this stage, to relabel their desired way of thinking and practising (their new theory of practice). It is important that the new labelling captures the person's own new understanding of their experience, using language that has emerged from their own reflections.

What contributors to this book were asked to address

Contributors were asked to describe the model they used (including its theoretical design and practical implementation) and, where appropriate, to comment on how it differs from the Fook and Gardner (2007) approach. Where possible, they have also tried to give a sense of the kinds of assumptions about practice that have emerged from participants' reflections, and to include the results of any formal evaluations they have conducted on the critical reflection process itself. Lastly they have included any personal observations about its use, especially in relation to the specific organisational contexts in which the reflection has been implemented. In this way, we have tried to include several types of data in each chapter: personal reflections, practical descriptions, research findings and observational material. We hope that each chapter, and the book as a whole, makes a contribution to the practical theorising of critical reflection, in particular its development and use in particular organisational settings.

Organisation of the book

The book is organised under four headings: professional practice; supervision and management; research; and education. These headings reflect the main ways in which we have found our critical reflection model has been used.

The case examples range over several different countries: Israel, Norway, Australia, the UK and Canada. They are also deliberately drawn from many different fields of practice. Our aim was to give as diverse a flavour as possible of the ways in which the model of critical reflection has been used and developed.

In the first section, the focus is on practice in particular fields: palliative care in Ireland (McLoughlin and McGilloway); in Australia, mental health (Gardner) and community development (Thomson); and also more generic usages, including connections with concepts of spirituality (Gardner). The second section focuses on uses in supervision, and includes examples from statutory work in the UK (Ferguson; Baker); the health sector in Australia (Gardner and Taalman); and social work student supervision (Lynne Allan). The final chapter in this section (Hearne) focuses on the use of critical reflection from a manager's perspective.

The third section, on the uses for research purposes, details three very different ways of using critical reflection as a research methodology. The first is written by a Norwegian researcher (Askeland) working in Ethiopia, using the model to develop an understanding of local culture and knowledge in Ethiopian social work. The chapter by Canadian Janet Allen details a modified use of the critical reflection model to research the use of spirituality; and Morley reflects on the use of the model to understand and change practice in sexual assault in Australia.

The section on teaching includes contributions from programmes in Israel (Savaya), Canada (Baikie et al.) and Australia (Delany and Watkin; Giles and Pockett).

The book closes with a chapter drawing together the main themes that have arisen about the practice of critical reflection in different settings and organisational contexts, and the implications for further theoretical and practical development of the model.

References

Boud, D. (2010) 'Relocating reflection in the context of practice', in Bradbury, H., Frost, N., Kilminster, S. and Zukas, M. (eds), *Beyond Reflective Practice*, London: Routledge, 25–36.

Boud, D., Cressey, P. and Docherty, P. (eds) (2006) *Productive Reflection at Work*, London: Routledge.

Boud, D., Keogh, R. and Walker, D. (1985) *Reflection: Turning Experience into Learning*, London: Kogan Page.

Brookfield, S. (1995) *Becoming a Critically Reflective Teacher*, San Francisco: Jossey-Bass.

——(2005) *The Power of Critical Theory*, San Francisco: Jossey-Bass.

Dewey, J. (1933) *How We Think*, Boston: Heath.

Fenwick, T. (2000) 'Expanding conceptions of experiential learning', *Adult Education Quarterly*, 50(4): 133–56.

Flyvberg, B. (2000) *Making Social Science Matter*, Cambridge: Cambridge University Press.

Fook, J. (2002) *Social Work: Critical Theory and Practice*, London: Sage.

——(2010) 'Beyond reflective practice: reworking the "critical" in critical reflection', in Bradbury, H., Frost, N., Kilminster, S. and Zukas, M. (eds), *Beyond Reflective Practice*, London: Routledge, 37–51.

——(2011) 'Developing critical reflection as a research method', in Higgs, J., Titchen, A., Horsfall, D. and Bridges, D. (eds), *Creative Spaces for Qualitative Researching*, Sense Publishers, Rotterdam, 55–64.

——(2012) 'Creating spaces for critically reflective groups', *Social Work with Groups*.

Fook, J. and Askeland, G.A. (2006) 'The "critical" in critical reflection', in White, S., Fook, J. and Gardner, F. (eds), *Critical Reflection in Health and Social Care*, Maidenhead: Open University Press, 40–53.

Fook, J. and Gardner, F. (2007) *Practising Critical Reflection: A Resource Handbook*, Maidenhead: Open University Press.

Fook, J. and Kellehear, A. (2010) 'Using critical reflection to support health promotion goals in palliative care', *Journal of Palliative Care*, 26(4): 295–302.

Fook, J., White, S. and Gardner, F. (2006) 'Critical reflection: a review of contemporary literature and understandings', in White, S., Fook, J. and Gardner, F. (eds), *Critical Reflection in Health and Social Care*, Maidenhead: Open University Press.

Gardner, F. (2011) *Critical Spirituality: A Holistic Approach to Contemporary Practice*, Farnham: Ashgate.

Gould, N. and Baldwin, M. (eds) (2004) *The Learning Organisation and Reflective Practice*, Aldershot: Ashgate.

Hoyrup, S. (2004) 'Reflection as a core process in organizational learning', *Journal of Workplace Learning*, 16(8): 442–54.

Humphrey, C. (2009) 'By the light of the Tao', *European Journal of Social Work*, 12(3): 377–90.

Hunt, C. (2010) 'A step too far: from professional reflective practice to spirituality', in Bradbury, H., Frost, N., Kilminster, S. and Zukas, M. (eds), *Beyond Reflective Practice*, London: Routledge, 155–69.

Johns, C. (2005) 'Balancing the winds', *Reflective Practice*, 6(1): 67–84.

Kolb, D.A. (1984) *Experiential Learning*, Englewood Cliffs, NJ: Prentice Hall.

Mezirow, J. and Associates (2000) *Learning as Transformation*, San Francisco: Jossey-Bass.

Munro, E. (2011) *The Munro Review of Child Protection: Final Report*, London: The Stationery Office.

Napier, L. and Fook, J. (2000) *Breakthroughs in Practice*, London: Whiting & Birch.

Norrie, C., Hammond, J., D'Avray, L., Collington, V. and Fook, J. (2012) 'Doing it differently? A review of literature on teaching reflective practice across health and social care professions', *Reflective Practice*, May, 1–14, DOI: 10.1080/14623943. 2012.670628.

Polkinghorne, D. (2004) *Practice and the Human Sciences*, New York: State University of New York Press.

Reynolds, M. and Vince, R. (eds) (2004) *Organizing Reflection*, Aldershot: Ashgate.

Ruch, G. (2005) 'Relationship-based and reflective practice', *Child and Family Social Work*, 10: 111–23.

——(2007) 'Reflective practice in contemporary child care social work: the role of containment', *British Journal of Social Work*, 37: 659–80.

——(2009) 'Identifying the "critical" in a relationship-based model of reflection', *European Journal of Social Work*, 12(3): 349–62.

Schön, D. (1983) *The Reflective Practitioner: How Professionals Think in Action*, New York: Basic Books.

Taylor, C. (2006) 'Practising reflexivity: narrative, reflection and the moral order', in White, S., Fook, J. and Gardner, F. (eds), *Critical Reflection in Health and Social Care*, Maidenhead: Open University Press, 73–88.

Taylor, C. and White, S. (2000) *Practising Reflexivity in Health and Social Welfare*, Buckingham: Open University Press.

Section 1

Critical reflection in professional practice

2 Unsettling assumptions around death, dying and palliative care

A practical approach

Kathleen McLoughlin and Sinéad McGilloway

Introduction

> Palliative care is an approach that improves the quality of life of patients and their families facing the problems associated with life-threatening illness, through the prevention and relief of suffering by means of early identification and impeccable assessment and treatment of pain and other problems, physical, psychosocial and spiritual.
>
> (WHO, 2002)

Despite the widely acknowledged benefits of early referral to palliative care (e.g. Teno and Ward, 2004), there is considerable evidence that many patients who could benefit from palliative care services are not referred in a timely manner and miss the opportunity to benefit from the health-promoting aspects of the service as they face the end of life. Referral to, and uptake of, palliative care services remains typically low (Casarett et al., 2005), and patients are often referred to services only in the final days of life. Thus many patients may make this important transition with just hours or days to live, and for some that transition might never occur.

The barriers to palliative care referral have been widely reported. There is considerable fear and stigma associated with palliative care services, most likely due to their association with death and dying. This fear and stigma is evident in patients contemplating referral, their families, the general public, and often also the health professionals who are the gatekeepers to palliative care (McLoughlin and McGilloway, 2011). Arguably, therefore, it is crucial that health professionals are offered an opportunity to critically reflect on their assumptions around palliative care, and to take time to explore their feelings toward death and dying, in a safe, facilitated environment. As part of a doctoral study, the authors developed a one-day course for health professionals entitled 'Working with death, dying and palliative care' (McLoughlin and McGilloway, 2011) utilising the Fook and Gardner (2007) model of critical reflection. The model was used as a basis to guide participants' learning during the workshop, whilst participants' thoughts and personal constructs around death, dying and palliative care were also examined utilising the repertory grid technique (Kelly, 1955).

This chapter explores the use of the Fook and Gardner (2007) model in the development of this innovative course and explains the rationale for adapting the model to suit the needs of the education programme and the target audience. With the permission of one course participant, a critical incident and learning scenario from the critical reflection process is presented here. The application of the rep grid technique to the critical incident description is also described. Further opportunities for the utilisation of critical reflection as a tool in palliative care education and health-promoting palliative care (Kellehear, 1999) are discussed.

This is my story

As part of a study to determine attitudes toward palliative care across a number of key groups, one-to-one interviews were conducted with health professionals who were in a position to refer patients to palliative care (McLoughlin and McGilloway, 2011). The findings from these interviews highlighted the important influence of personal and professional experience on attitudes toward palliative care; the use of personal and professional stories in the accounts of health professionals was extremely common. All health professionals, at some point in their interview, referred to their own story of death, dying, loss or care that had touched their life. For many, this was the death of a parent; for one, of a child. Sometimes the reference to personal experience was used solely to highlight a point. For example:

> 'It must be awful to die in pain – my father died a few years ago, he just dropped dead. It was such a shock but looking back at least we know he didn't really suffer' [P5].

The remaining participants seemed to dwell on their tale of loss, and moved away from the interview topic, explaining in great detail the circumstances surrounding the death, their feelings at the time and now. One participant discussed their personal loss for over 20 minutes, and two became quite emotional whilst speaking. Their personal tale certainly seemed to have a powerful influence on their professional practice, understanding and attitude toward palliative care, as highlighted below:

> 'I don't think education influences attitudes toward palliative care, it is shaped by previous experience of those we have cared for who have died. I lost my father in 1999 and now I understand how the dying process works and what it is like to be left behind, so that has influenced my practice and changed the way I deal with family members now' [P3].

The health professionals' stories all had relatively positive outcomes, and we explored the effects on practice, understanding and attitudes toward palliative care for those whose experience may not have been so positive.

In addition to personal stories, each health professional also voluntarily referred to a patient story as an example to illustrate their points. Interestingly, most of the patient stories discussed by health professionals were used to indicate a difficult or complex case, or an area where systems/services had failed. For example:

> 'I was visiting Mary for several months and every time I called she told me she was absolutely fine. After a few weeks, her daughter called me, daily sometimes, telling me that her mother was in so much pain ... but she just wouldn't admit it to me ... crazy' [P4].

Participants often went on to reflect how they might have done things differently:

> 'Looking back, I should have realised more quickly how depressed he was. The minute I mentioned it to the consultant, a referral was made to the mental health team in X' [P3].

Health professionals seemed very comfortable with utilising these patient stories or case studies during the interviews and critically reflecting on them (albeit at a very basic level); this led us to consider how utilising and processing individual personal and professional stories might serve as a potentially powerful educational tool to enable health professionals to explore their own attitudes toward, and experience of, death, dying, loss and care. The use of stories and case studies is common in palliative and gerontology education provision (Kirkpatrick and Brown, 2004) and the use of reflection is also encouraged. Interestingly, the tendency to discuss 'negative-outcome' patient stories to reference points made in their interviews regarding palliative care led us to consider whether the use of critical reflection (Fook and Gardner, 2007) in palliative education could prove particularly beneficial. Fook and Kellehear (2010) suggest that critical reflection is a useful method for learning about practice experience in palliative care, and is particularly helpful in that it includes an emotional element, thereby allowing health professionals an opportunity to process emotionally rich critical incidents that may have personal and/or professional origins.

Such a framework was considered appropriate because it involves exploring the underlying assumptions that people (in this case health professionals) make about the situations (in this case patients) they experience. This can be useful for health professionals as it allows them to explore fundamental assumptions they make about their practice and provides a 'space' to enable a reworking of these (if necessary). The Fook and Gardner (2007) model had particular appeal given that it is well documented, clear and accessible. The model is designed for use in a group setting and therefore offers an opportunity for participants to learn, not only from critically reflecting on their own incident, but also from engaging in and questioning incidents described by other participants.

Working with death, dying and palliative care

A face-to-face, one-day workshop was developed for qualified healthcare professionals who were in a position to refer cancer patients to specialist palliative care services. In an earlier phase of this study, it was found that, whilst experience, case studies and personal attitudes or constructs were important indicators of health professionals' attitudes toward palliative care, there were other factors that also need to be considered. For this reason, the course was loosely based on a model of critical reflection (Fook and Gardner, 2007) and was designed within a health-promoting palliative care (Kellehear, 1999) and adult learning framework. The main aim of the workshop was to reduce health professionals' fear and stigma associated with death, dying, loss and care through the medium of an adapted approach to critical reflection (Fook and Gardner, 2007). This approach aims to engage participants in open and honest discussion about death and dying, and the potential benefits of palliative care, through the analysis of critical incidents submitted in advance by workshop participants. A didactic element was also provided as part of the workshop to enable participants to consider and understand the aim and purpose of palliative care and to obtain further information regarding palliative care service availability and options. A session within the proposed workshop was dedicated to reflection on one's own mortality using a guided visualisation process. A communication skills session was also included as part of the workshop.

A participants' handbook was developed to outline the structure and purpose of the workshop to prospective participants. This contained pre-course activities for completion and outlined the structure of the workshop and guidelines for potential participants. It also included advice that, if participants had experienced a significant personal bereavement during the previous 12 months, they should not take part in the course due to the potentially emotional impact of some of the issues raised therein.

Critical incidents and assumptions – a note

Interestingly, 'critical incident' and 'assumption', as used by Fook and Gardner (2007), were terms that health professionals (who were not necessarily familiar with the theory) reviewing the material for the workshop struggled with. In the current climate, critical incidents are usually referred to in a health service environment within a quality and risk framework, where critical incidents are reported as near-miss events or injuries as part of clinical indemnity schemes and a culture of health and safety. This led to some confusion and an overly negative or traumatic connotation when the term was used in the workshop. Participants seemed to feel that it was necessary to write about a time when something went wrong, or when harm occurred, and as a result there was a risk that they may have felt they were going to be exposed as poor practitioners in some way. It was therefore very important to explain and reassure participants as to exactly what was required of them. Likewise, the term 'assumption' was questioned rather defensively by some participants; one participant felt that the facilitators were 'questioning her intelligence'. The learning here is that the model, when applied across settings, needs to consider the language and frames of reference of potential participants, and may need to soften or define the terms, as outlined in the activity instructions below.

Generating the story for analysis

In advance of the workshop, participants were asked to complete the following activity (adapted from Fook and Gardner, 2007).

Pre-course activity 1

This activity is central to the course. Please think of a situation from your past or current professional work (or personal life, if you feel it is relevant to your professional practice). We will use the description of this situation in the workshop as a basis for reflection on your practice.

> Think of a time when a patient you cared for could/should have been referred to specialist palliative care, but for some reason was not, or was referred to the service very late. The more specific and focused you can be the better.

Here is what we would like to know:

- why this patient situation was selected by you (why did this one stick out for you?)
- the context/background of the patient's situation (a simple description of any background the group might need to know to make the incident meaningful)
- the actual situation (a simple description of events, your thoughts and feelings (if relevant), behaviours/actions, what was said).

In choosing your patient situation, please keep in mind the following.

- Confidentiality – protecting other people's reputations, identities. You will be presenting to a group of people, some of whom you may know. It is important to protect, as far as possible, the confidentiality of anyone else who may have been involved with your patient. If you feel that discussing a patient from your current practice may jeopardise this, you may choose a situation from the past, or you may change any identifying information.
- Your own preparedness for exposure. Please choose a situation you are prepared to discuss in a group of people (some of whom you may know well). You need to be comfortable with divulging some aspects of your thinking and practice, which may also be personal. Sometimes this kind

of reflection unearths aspects of ourselves of which we were not previously aware, so we need to be prepared to expose some of this. On the other hand, this course is not about personal exposure purely for the sake of it, and there may be some things which you would prefer to keep private.

• The patient you choose is entirely your decision; however, the situation must involve a patient who could/should have been referred to specialist palliative care, but for some reason was not, or was referred to the service very late. It is important that you choose a scenario from which you feel you can learn something by critically reflecting on it in a short period.

An example of a critical incident generated by a course participant (Mary) is outlined below. This is used throughout the chapter as a case study. To protect confidentiality and anonymity, all names have been changed.

Mary's critical incident

I have chosen this situation as it is complex due to the relationships involved, and the issue of urgency was very real and posed challenges to working with the patient and family. Although there was limited time for social work intervention before the patient's death, there has been a considerable amount of contact since. This contact has been challenging as the family seem to have unrealistic expectations of what interventions or support can be offered.

The patient was a 35-year-old woman who had been diagnosed with breast cancer approximately two years before her death. The referral to palliative care came from her public health nurse [PHN] who was requesting social work support for the patient's eight-year-old daughter, and also an exploration of what memory work could be done with the patient. The patient was not open to nursing or medical input from the hospice team as she had not received any conventional treatment for her illness; she had attended an alternative therapist and was still hopeful of cure. At the point of referral, the PHN had stated that this lady was very unwell and that her prognosis was poor. She was symptomatic in terms of pain from a wound, but refused input. The patient's father had died two years prior from cancer, and had been cared for by the homecare team. Her mother was alive and helped to care for her. She had one sister, who suffered from bipolar disorder. She was separated from her daughter's father.

The patient agreed to meet with a social worker, and a colleague of mine (who I supervised) met with her. She made a tentative start on a memory book about her life to leave for her daughter. The social worker also met the patient's daughter twice to try to explore her understanding of the illness. At the time, we were both conscious of how tentative this contact was, and that the social worker had to be careful in her approach in case the patient ended the contact and perhaps withdrew from the service entirely. We had a sense that she was suffering significant pain, but we felt helpless as she had refused GP and home care team intervention. We felt this was a shame, as it was very possible that she could have been made so much more comfortable.

She did eventually concede to accepting the home care team and was admitted to the hospice for symptom control. She died the day after admission. Everyone was shocked by her death. The patient's daughter was, by this time, living with her father and paternal grandmother. Relations were not good between them and the patient's mother and sister, so there were tensions evident when the child was brought to see her mother's body. The social worker facilitated this event. Contact with the little girl and her father for bereavement support continued after the patient's death. Contact with the patient's own family was more chaotic and sporadic – they had asked me to intervene with the child's father regarding access issues. Relationships between them broke down completely and they pursued a legal route to gain access to the child.

Fundamentally, I felt very sorry for them that it had to come to this, and that this little girl had lost her mum, but also her grandmother and her aunt too.

Using the repertory grid technique

The 'Working with death, dying and palliative care' workshop was used on this occasion as part of a research study, and one of the measures used in the study was the rep grid. Whilst the development of a rep grid based on a narrative or story has been used before in the field of death and dying, developing a rep grid specifically from a critical incident is unique. The rep grid is a technique for identifying the ways in which a person construes (interprets/gives meaning to) his or her experience, and is a tool developed to support Kelly's (1955) theory of personal construct psychology (PCP).

According to PCP (Kelly, 1955), each person employs a system of many bipolar personal constructs, each of which serves to organise and attribute meaning to some portion of the world. A construct is defined as 'a way in which some things are alike and different from others' (Jankowicz, 2004). The 'things' in this definition are referred to as elements of the construct. An element may refer to a concrete object, person and event, or to an abstract process or concept. The theory holds that a person's system of constructs is organised in a hierarchical fashion, with relationships of superordination and subordination among constructs (Kelly, 1955). Among the most superordinate constructs in the system are the core constructs. These are especially important as they are at the centre of a person's existence and personal identity, and any change in them will disturb the person deeply. If a person's identity and understanding of the world is challenged, he/she is said to experience threat (of death, in the context of this study), which impairs their ability to predict events in the world accurately. The person becomes aware of a need to undertake systematic change in order to re-predict events accurately. There are degrees of threat according to the extent to which a person's construct system has been challenged. The more superordinate the construct, the greater the portion of the system being challenged (Winter, 1992).

We will now explore how the rep grid may be potentially beneficial to critical reflection.

Excavation of the elements

The rep grid technique and the concept of elements and constructs were used by the researcher (KMcL), who reviewed Mary's critical incident scenario and identified the key people or elements relative to the timeframes in the incident as follows:

- self at the time of intervention with the patient/family (3)
- self after the intervention with the patient/family (4)
- your colleague (5)
- patient before referral (6)
- patient at the time of death (7)
- patient on referral to social work (8)
- patient's daughter before the patient died (12)
- patient's daughter viewing mother's body (13)
- patient's daughter now (14)
- patient's mother before patient died (15)
- patient's mother when patient died (16)
- patient's mother now (17)
- patient's sister before patient died (18)
- patient's sister at the time of death (19)
- patient's sister now (20)
- patient's partner before patient's death (21)
- patient's partner at the time of death (22)
- patient's partner now (23)

In addition to these participant-generated elements, other elements that were standard across all participants' grids (for the research process) were included as follows:

- ideal self (1)
- self now (2)
- a patient receiving non-conventional treatment for cancer (9)
- a palliative care patient with a cancer diagnosis (10)
- a patient receiving conventional treatment for cancer (11)
- a dying person (24)
- a person receiving palliative care (25)

Digging out the constructs

The elements were entered into a grid (see Figure 2.1) and each element label from the list above was written onto a piece of card. The cards were presented to the participant in triads as follows:

A: Ideal self – self now – self after interaction with family
B: The one from A that is different – self at the time patient accepted intervention – colleague
C: Patient before referral – Patient at time of death – Patient on referral to social work
D: Non conventional treatment for cancer – palliative care for cancer – conventional treatment for cancer
E: Patient's daughter (all 3)
F: Patient's mother (all 3)
G: Patient's sister (all 3)
H: Patient's husband (all 3)
I: Patient on referral to social work – dying person – person receiving palliative care

Upon presentation of each triad, the participant was asked to identify which two elements were alike and therefore different from the third. They were

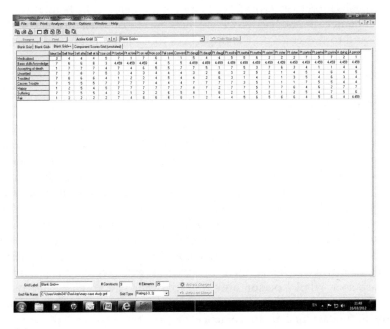

Figure 2.1

then asked to name what it was that made the two elements similar and what they considered to be the opposite of that. From this, a series of bipolar constructs emerged and were entered onto the grid (Figure 2.1). For example, on presentation of triad C, the participant identified that the patient before referral and on referral to social work was 'in denial and resistant' as opposed to 'accepting of death'. Participants then rated each element on each bipolar construct on a scale from 1 to 7 and the grid was populated (Figure 2.1).

The data from the grid were then entered into IDIOGRID (a rep grid software analysis program) for principal component analysis (Figure 2.1) and graphical representation. For ease of interpretation, the elements have been recoded on the graph using numbers aligned to the numbers in brackets in the element list. The graph considers only components 1 and 2 given the two-dimensional constraints here.

Knowing what matters

A total of 79.6% of the total variance in Mary's grid was accounted for by the first three components, thereby suggesting that these were central to her conceptualisation of this situation. Component 1 (48.2% total variance) was associated with **psychological wellbeing**, with high loading of constructs around happiness, peacefulness, feeling settled and comfortable – see horizontal axis on Figure 2.2. Component 2 (17.3% total variance) focused on **medicalisation** (see vertical axis), and component 3 (14.1% total variance) on **acceptance.** Immediately, we are now aware of what matters to Mary with regard to this case study and, perhaps more importantly, with regard to caring for patients and their family at the end of life.

Who matters the most?

Ordination is a measure of the ordinal position and meaningfulness of constructs in a rep grid (Landfield and Cannell, 1988). A high ordination score for a given construct indicates that it is superordinate or more meaningful when compared with other constructs in the grid. Mary had high ordination scores on the elements associated with the patient at the time of referral and the patient's mother at the time of death. The elements associated with Mary herself were the lowest-scoring in terms of ordination, and this was particularly interesting as, during the grid process, Mary seemed to refer to herself as a 'social worker' and herself as 'Mary' when rating self elements on the constructs; she seemed to struggle with regard to providing a response as a 'whole' person and appeared reluctant to share her real self with the researcher. The notion of placing the patient and family at the centre is fundamental to the practice of palliative care and therefore it is fitting that Mary places more importance on these elements. In looking at

3/16/2012 (12:15:32 PM)

PCA (no rotation) for Blank Grid++
Axis Range: -1.07 to   1.07

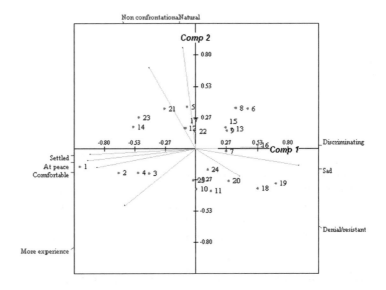

Figure 2.2

the grid and how Mary construes herself now (2), her ideal self (1), herself at the time of referral (3), and herself after the patient died (4), the grid highlights that Mary remains stable with regard to component 2, seeing herself almost mid-way between medicalised and natural view of death (slightly more medical), with more variation on psychological distress over time illustrating that, as time has passed, she has become more accepting of the situation with regard to the case study (and possibly with palliative care practice as a social worker or life as Mary). There is little distance between the self and the ideal self, suggesting that Mary is well adjusted and has high self-esteem.

The information obtained from the grid and the elicitation process are useful in helping the facilitator to focus on certain aspects in the critical reflection workshop, thereby enabling the participant – in this case, Mary – to access more quickly the deeper issues. For example, what assumptions did Mary make about herself as 'Mary the social worker' and as 'Mary the person'? Working in palliative care, where issues of death, dying, loss and care have a personal and professional relevance, what assumptions do we make about dealing with those issues, and how healthy is the 'split' that Mary has created? Had Mary's self-esteem been low, the facilitator may have chosen to focus on ordinance as part of the critical reflection process; for example, what assumptions does Mary make about herself if she always places the greatest importance on the patient and family?

Questions ... questions ... questions ...

The grid shows significant distance between Mary and her colleague (5) whom she was supervising at the time of the incident. This may be worthy of greater deconstruction during the workshop.

- What assumptions did Mary make about her colleague?
- How did these assumptions affect Mary's feelings and practice about the case?
- How might these assumptions have affected the outcome for the patient and family?

Comparing the patient in this case study and Mary's constructs of a typical dying person, we see that the patient was slightly more distressed and less medicalised. What assumptions does Mary make about patients who choose not to pursue the medicalised models of care and seek to engage in more natural practice around death? The grid enables us to pose many questions about the critical incident that are potentially more focused than might otherwise be the case using the standard Fook and Gardner approach.

Making the link between grids and critical reflection

The use of the rep grid offers a potentially very interesting pre-course activity for facilitators that enables a greater insight into participants' construct systems prior to the main group session, thereby enabling them to determine how the participant perceives themself in relation to those in the incident, and to explore who and what matters most to the participant regarding that incident. The use of the grid may also offer a useful validation of the critical reflection process whereby a facilitator can explore the juxtaposition of the emerging issues in the group with the individual manifestations through the grid process. The grid offers many potential questions that might prove to be useful prompts for the facilitator to 'dig deep' as part of the critical reflection process during the relatively early stages of the workshop. It also offers a tangible visual aid with which both participants and facilitator can work to compose questions and explore complex relationships between people in the case study, and to construct systems around a particular topic. The grid also offers a possible means of evaluating Fook and Gardner's model of critical reflection if implemented on a pre/post-course basis, by providing both a qualitative and quantitative measure of change in participants over time.

Where to next?

The rep grid technique and critical reflection offer a potentially useful basis for the development of interventions for health professionals and people living with advanced life-limiting illness that would contribute to much-needed changes in the 'death-defying' culture that appears to be predominant. Whilst Kellehear (1984) has argued against the 'denial of death' thesis *per se*, he suggests that the development of health-promoting palliative care interventions that include health and death education is vital to enable society to engage in issues associated with death, dying, loss and care, and ultimately to change behaviours and practice. The use of rep grids, coupled with critical reflection, offers a potentially promising means of shaking up our construct systems and unsettling our assumptions around end-of-life care.

References

Casarett, D.J. (2000) 'Are special guidelines needed for palliative care research?', *Journal of Pain and Symptom Management*, 20(2): 130–39.

Casarett, D., Crowley, R., Stevenson, C., Xie, S. and Teno, J. (2005) 'Making difficult decisions about hospice enrollment: what do patients and families want to know?', *Journal of the American Geriatric Society*, 53(2): 249–54.

Fook, J. and Gardner, F. (2007) *Practising Critical Reflection: A Resource Handbook*, Maidenhead: Open University Press.

Fook, J. and Kellehear, A. (2010) 'Using critical reflection to support health promotion goals in palliative care', *Journal of Palliative Care*, 26(4): 295–302.

Jankowicz, D. (2004) *The Easy Guide to Repertory Grids*, Chichester: Wiley.

Kellehear, A. (1984) 'Are we a death-denying society? A sociological review', *Social Science and Medicine*, 18(9): 713–21.

——(1999) *Health Promoting Palliative Care*, Melbourne: Oxford University Press.

Kelly, G.A. (1955) *The Psychology of Personal Constructs*, New York: Norton.

Kirkpatrick, M.K. and Brown, S. (2004) 'Narrative pedagogy: teaching geriatric content with stories and the "Make a Difference" project', *Nursing Education Perspective*, 25(4): 183–87.

Landfield, A.W. and Cannell, J.E. (1988) 'Ways of assessing functionally independent construction, meaningfulness, and construction in hierarchy', in Mancuso, J.C. and Shaw, M.L.G. (eds), *Cognition and Personal Structure: Computer Access and Analysis*, New York: Praeger, 67–90.

McLoughlin, K. (2011) 'Identifying and changing attitudes toward palliative care: an exploratory study', PhD thesis, National University of Ireland Maynooth.

McLoughlin, K. and McGilloway, S. (2008) 'Health promotion in palliative care: identifying and responding to attitudinal barriers to service use', *National Institute of Health Sciences Research Bulletin*, 4: 3.

——(2011) *Working with Death and Dying: Participants' Handbook*, National University of Ireland Maynooth.

Teno, J. and Ward, N.S. (2004) 'Family perspectives on end-of-life care at the last place of care', *JAMA*, 291(1): 88–93.

WHO (2002) 'WHO definition of palliative care', Geneva: World Health Organization, www.who.int/cancer/palliative/definition/en

Winter, D.A. (1992) *Personal Construct Psychology in Clinical Practice*, London: Routledge.

3 Integrating spirituality and critical reflection

Toward critical spirituality

Fiona Gardner

Introduction

This chapter explores my interest in integrating spirituality with critical reflection, in two ways. I begin by identifying how spirituality and critical reflection are currently perceived and how each can contribute to the other in what I have called 'critical spirituality'. Secondly, I use a particular example typical of my experience in running workshops focusing on spirituality that is underpinned by critical reflection theory. This example explores the reactions of a small training group to an exercise in a workshop, and illustrates the potential value of a critically spiritual approach to training and practice.

Part one: spirituality and critical reflection – the potential for integration

Spirituality is increasingly of interest to professionals in health and social care settings. White (2006: 43) says 'Spirituality can be understood broadly as a concern with transcendent aspects of life such as meaning, purpose and hope, suggesting a relevance to many issues that are pertinent to health care teams.' The literature suggests that many professionals recognise the need to include spirituality in their practice, but feel inadequately trained to do so (Haynes et al., 2007). What is also agreed is that spirituality is hard to define. Rumbold (2002: 9) suggests that spirituality is named differently in different disciplines and lacks a clear, generally accepted definition, but has become a way 'of asserting personal authority and identity in the face of scientific authority that neglected the subjective, relational and transcendent aspects of identity'.

The need to include spirituality is seen as particularly clear in such areas of health and social care as loss and grief, responding to disasters, palliative care, rehabilitation and chronic illness, where people are facing issues either of mortality or of the need to make decisions that will make significant difference to their lives (Abbas and Panjwani, 2008). However, there are many other ways in which the issue of spirituality is raised for professionals. Some writers would argue that there is more interest in religion and spirituality in general, particularly in developing your own expression of spirituality (Forman, 2004; Kavanagh, 2007). Others suggest that increased migration has meant that workers are confronted with clients for whom religious beliefs are a significant part of how they live (Stirling et al., 2010). Issues connected to religion and spirituality can emerge in any health and social care field, including child protection (Gilligan, 2009); work with asylum seekers (Ní Raghallaigh, 2011); in aged care (MacKinlay, 2008); and in mental health (Martin, 2009).

Including the spiritual remains, however, a contested area. Partly, this is for obvious reasons: spiritual and religious differences generate conflict within families and communities, and between nations. There are also justified concerns about practitioners imposing their spiritual values on others or simply being insufficiently aware of how their own assumptions and values influence their practice in unhelpful ways (Helmeke and Sori, 2006; McCurdy, 2008). Winslow and Wehtje-Winslow (2007: 63) remind health care workers to be mindful of patients' vulnerability and 'ethical boundaries of spiritual care'. Hoffman et al. (2005) worry that therapists assume their own spiritual experience is enough training for working with clients on theirs. On the other hand, not including spirituality can mean clients feel that what matters and helps them is not recognised (Nichols and Hunt, 2011). Wong and Vinsky (2009) indicate the importance of recognising that it can be religion that matters to individuals and communities. Gray and Lovat (2008: 160) point out that 'At the heart of social work's aversion to religion lies its fear of absolutism and moralism, but religion need not be so. In fact, spirituality can just as easily be a haven for fixed thinking and dogmatic beliefs.' It is also fair to say that absolutism and moralism can apply equally to other beliefs, such as political views or simply even beliefs about how things should be done (Canda and Furman, 2010).

These concerns support the need for including spirituality in training for professional practice, but also the need for, and value of, including the capacity to reflect on practice. White's (2006) research included meeting with a multi-professional team at a palliative care centre to explore how spirituality could inform their practice. She concluded that reflective practice was an important way to explore spirituality, with the group providing a 'safe space' for learning. While there are variations in definitions of reflective practice and critical reflection (Fook et al., 2006) research on the inclusion of spirituality in practice generally supports the need for a critically reflective approach, the combining of self-reflection with awareness of cultural and social context (Swinton, 2001; McSherry, 2007).

The Fook and Gardner (2007) approach to critical reflection outlined in chapter 1 is particularly useful for considering the ways in which the two threads – spirituality and critical reflection – can complement and strengthen each other. This is perhaps most obvious in the linked use of critical social theory related to how social assumptions and values are internalised and expressed, as well as commitment to action for social justice change, individually and collectively. From a spiritual perspective, liberation theologians and activists document a significant history of engaging with the ideas and 'praxis' of critical social theory. Essentially, liberation theology has emerged from religious traditions, and makes connections between what is personal and what is political in order to achieve a socially just society for those who experience oppression (Lartey, 2003). What is particularly helpful here is its exploration of power and the clarity of its social justice approach. Liberation theologies also make explicit that strategies of 'power over', such as violence and abuse in the name of religion or spirituality, are not acceptable. In exploring how at least some liberation theology groups might work more closely together, Ruether (2006: 328) suggests a new, combined 'ecofeminist theology' that 'calls us to repent of power over others and to reclaim power within and power with one another … This is a vision of life energy that calls us all into life-giving community from many strands of tradition, culture and history.' The importance of community expressed in liberation theology is often seen as one of the distinctive and valued features of religious traditions (Heelas and Woodhead, 2005).

A liberation theology approach, like the post-modern theory underlying critical reflection, values diversity and affirms the right of individuals to be able to express themselves in the context of their preferred spiritual or religious tradition. Its diversity is one of the strengths and complexities of the current liberation theology movement, with groups focused on the oppression of those who are – for example – experiencing poverty (Rowland, 1999), women (Ruether, 1985; Gross, 2009), lesbian (Kamitsuka, 2007), Muslim and homosexual (al-Haqq Kugle, 2010), and those who experience a combination of ways of feeling marginalised or excluded in a particular culture, such as being gay, black and Christian (Sneed, 2010). Berry (2009) advocates 'ecological spirituality'. The richness of writing from liberation theology provides useful examples about actively valuing diversity and related community change. Sneed's experience is of being black and gay in a Christian church where being black is seen as the primary issue of difference. He argues for greater complexity of critical thinking, and a focus on the question 'What makes for human happiness and fulfilment?' (Sneed, 2010: 181).

Another aspect of valuing difference from comes from writing about differences in a person's 'spiritual journey' or pathway, with an expectation that this will change over time. Interestingly, such writers acknowledge the importance of movement towards a more critically reflective approach to life, including spiritual understanding (Fowler, 1981; Wilber, 1997). Trelfa suggests that, for students, it can help to name such changes as loss of certainty or 'calling' as part of 'normal' change over time on a spiritual journey. She suggests that reflective practice, like spiritual faith, provides a dependable life space that is 'profound, ultimate, and stable no matter what happens at the level of the immediate event' (Trelfa, 2005: 208).

A reflective or critically reflective approach to spirituality is advocated in developing cultural competence for practice (Holloway and Moss, 2010; Hodge, 2011). Others identify the need to identify underlying assumptions and beliefs about spirituality and religion that may have an impact on practice (Gilligan, 2009), as well as the capacity to be reflexive: to be able to understand that how you perceive others may not be how they perceive you (Gardner, 2011). There is also clearly a connection to the increasing literature on ethics and morality or integrity (Banks, 2008, 2010); ethics and moral courage (Murray, 2010); and perceptions of conscience (Gustafsson et al., 2010; Laabs, 2011), which link questions of meaning and values with the need for reflection or critical reflection to help manage the complexities of practice.

Another benefit of making explicit the links between spirituality and critical reflection is the expectation of working holistically. Some practice disciplines have been better than others at including the spiritual in practice: in nursing, for example, there is a significant body of literature, perhaps because nurses are more likely to confront life-and-death issues. Including the spiritual with critical reflection further validates the focus on meaning at a fundamental level. In critical reflection, the aim is to unearth deeply held assumptions and values; a spiritual approach affirms the value of working with what really matters. Gray and Lovat (2008: 157), writing for social workers, say 'whether one speaks of critical reflection or meditation, one is describing a process of heightening consciousness or awareness of one's own knowing'.

Using the language of meditation is a reminder of the value of a contemplative or 'being' state of mind in approaching reflective practice. Johns (2005), from a nursing background, affirms reflective practice as a 'way of being' connected to the mystical in religious traditions such as Buddhism. This awareness of a more contemplative or being attitude can generate more listening in critical reflection: a greater capacity to sit with the person rather than feeling compelled to act. Gray and Lovat combine this 'awareness of knowing' with critical theory in 'practical mysticism', 'which leads to an understanding of common values across religions resulting in praxis, practical action for good' (Gray and Lovat, 2008: 159).

This links, in religious terms, to being comfortable also with 'unknowing' or not knowing, being able to sit with uncertainty. Vernon (2007) expresses concern that religion may be perceived as being about certainty rather than what he perceives as more important: comfort with the unknowable and unknown. Relating this to practice suggests examples of being prepared to sit with people as they accept not knowing – such as when someone is seriously ill and it cannot be known what will happen. In critical reflection, the capacity to sit with another's 'not knowing' is also important: allowing exploration, rather than moving too quickly to seeking solutions.

Clarity about language helps: what definition of spirituality and religion is being used? I have combined spirituality and critical reflection in defining 'critical spirituality' as 'that which gives life meaning, including a sense of something beyond or greater than the self', but that also maintains awareness of the influence of history and social context (Gardner, 2011: 19). Such a definition has the benefit of being highly inclusive, applicable both to spirituality in its broadest sense and to religious practice. Such a definition can encourage professionals to see how spirituality can be included in their practice. Asking about meaning is something that is often lost in the busyness of organisational and client issues. Thinking about spirituality in this broader sense encourages standing back from the immediate, seeing what is happening in a more holistic way, and asking what really matters for client and worker.

Part two: integration spirituality and critical reflection in training – an example

The second part of this chapter explores the use of critical reflection in training related to working with spirituality. I have used material from two sets of workshops run through the Centre for Professional Development, Latrobe University, Australia. The first were one-day workshops titled 'Spirituality and work', developed in response to practitioners feeling they were expected to respond to 'spiritual' issues without knowing how. These workshops included reflecting on similarities and differences in spirituality and religion, the participants' own sense of the spiritual, and implications of including spirituality for practice.

The second set of workshops was a series of three-day training workshops for professionals and volunteers in palliative care and related settings, titled 'Spirituality/pastoral care in palliative care'. These were part of a pilot project responding to a health care survey suggesting that palliative care clients and their families did not have as much access to pastoral or spiritual care as they would have liked. After a consultation with local service providers, volunteers and community members, it was agreed that all those involved in palliative care ideally would develop sufficient skills to be able to respond to such issues, with referral to specialist pastoral care workers as needed. The aim was to equip participants for this role. Training included knowledge about spirituality and religion, encouraging awareness of one's own values and how these differ from other people's, practice in listening, ability to care for yourself, awareness of roles of others in the team, and consciousness of when to refer on (Gardner and Nolan, 2009). These workshops differed significantly in their primary aims from the critical reflection workshops of Fook and Gardner (2007), where participants came expecting to develop understanding of the theory and processes of critical reflection, to experience using the model and consider implications for practice.

However, the theory outlined in chapter 1, which underpins critical reflection, was used in developing the workshops. Because of their different and multiple aims, the underlying theory of critical reflection was not presented formally. Instead, theoretical ideas related to the historical and social context of religion and health care provided a direct link to the issues raised in postmodernism and critical social theory: considering the impact of dominant ways of thinking on individuals as well as communities. This provoked discussion about the influence of the broader social context that influenced participants as professionals and personally. For those in palliative care, attitudes to death and dying in the community clearly affected what was possible organisationally, and so how flexible individual staff felt their practice could be. They connected postmodern thinking about the dominant discourses about illness to the lack of power of clients – and often themselves in the health system; the tendency for clients to be seen as an illness rather than a whole person; the binaries of being healthy or ill, right or wrong. Participants identified how they internalised prevailing attitudes to spirituality and religion as well as health care for the dying, and how this might limit their creativity and flexibility.

Reflective practice and reflexivity were used in developing a series of exercises, again implicitly. The workshops were primarily experiential, a series of exercises that encouraged participants to explore their own and others' spirituality. This allowed for and encouraged the exploration of assumptions and values outlined in the first stage of the model. The feedback from these exercises was then used for second-stage applications: to consider implications for practice – changed assumptions as well as possible actions. Another difference from the model was that, rather than focusing on one specific incident, the participants brought a range of experiences for discussion, though they used a specific experience in relation to each exercise.

Those attending 'Spirituality and work' workshops generally came from the health field, particularly rehabilitation, acute health care, palliative care and community health; a small number were from education. Participants generally came because they felt there was a need to include spirituality in their practice, sometimes in response to changes in organisational expectations, and this was not included in professional training. Those attending the palliative care workshops either worked or volunteered in palliative care or in related agencies such as aged care settings, and also felt unprepared for including spirituality in their practice.

Critical reflection in training: Monica's and Teresa's experience

I will use a typical interaction from workshops to explore how the underlying theories and processes of critical reflection are used in this training to explore spirituality and its inclusion in practice. I have changed names and details to maintain confidentiality. The workshops all began by establishing a climate of 'critical acceptance' (Fook, Ryan and Hawkins, 2000: 230–31). In this exercise, participants had been asked to think about what they would want from professionals, from a spiritual perspective, if they were seriously ill or dying. The two women in this example both came from Catholic backgrounds. Monica was in her early fifties and had remained faithful to Catholicism all her life, finding it a source of great support in her work, particularly now as an acute care nurse in a Catholic hospital. Teresa, now in her thirties, rejected Catholicism in her late teens, partly because a gay friend felt unaccepted within the church community, and continued to feel hostile to Catholicism. She preferred 'open spirituality', a combination of meditation which she had learnt from both Christian and Buddhist traditions, the use of crystals and colours, and she had recently become interested in Wiccan spirituality. Teresa also worked in health care, as a palliative care nurse.

Monica and Teresa paired up to share their responses to what they would want from a professional if seriously ill or dying. Each felt considerably challenged by what the other said she would want – conceivably from each other, given their work roles. Monica said she could see Teresa physically recoil when she said she might ask Teresa to hand her a rosary and want support in saying it. Similarly, Teresa felt Monica was incredulous that she could want to hang crystals next to her hospital bed, and that Monica wasn't able to respond in any neutral, as opposed to positive, way to Wiccan healing practices. In reporting back to the larger group, both expressed their surprise and concern about how strongly and how negatively they had reacted to the other person and their preferences. They had perceived themselves as non-judgemental and accepting of difference, particularly in relation to spirituality in others. They were concerned about what this might mean for their practice with people they perceived as being more significantly different, such as those from Muslim or Jewish traditions. Other group members had varied experiences in their pairs: some had felt simply interested or fascinated by the similarities and differences that emerged, but they could all relate to what Monica and Teresa were saying.

Observations from the process

Typically, what emerged from the discussion that followed was:

The value of reflection and self awareness: the need to reflect critically on one's own assumptions and values

This exercise reinforced for all the participants the need to be aware of their own reactions and where they were coming from. There were, of course, assumptions and values that people wanted to affirm and that were common across the group – for example, that spirituality is an important aspect of people's lives and that spirituality should therefore be part of their professional practice.

Participants were at least surprised, and for some quite taken aback, by some of their underlying assumptions and values. Hearing from others in the group about where they were coming from confronted people very directly with different assumptions and values. This helped people clarify their own, and how they were similar to, or different from, others'. The value of reflection was reinforced by taking time to consider what was influencing a particular reaction – the mixture of personal and social/cultural history and values for each person.

Recognising the difference between their espoused values and values in action

This example demonstrated the difference between what Schön (1983) called espoused values – those participants thought they used – and those used in action. Theoretically, all participants would have affirmed 'celebrating diversity' in their practice. However, this example prompted the group to acknowledge a collective 'ouch' at a shared sense of 'but really my way is the better way'. Again, this reinforced building in reflection in practice to ensure a sense of openness to other ways.

Recognising the impact of assumptions on perceptions

Participants were also surprised by how they were perceived by others. The importance of understanding the complexities of reflexivity quickly became clear. Monica felt that Teresa saw her as a conservative Catholic, making assumptions about what her Catholicism meant for her, and its influence on her life and values, that were not how Monica perceived herself: 'Just because I use a rosary', she said, 'doesn't mean I agree with all of the policies of the Church'. She acknowledged that she also made assumptions about Teresa, based on her spirituality, that made it hard to see the person. Each was also conscious of feeling 'put in a box' by the other, so that everything they said confirmed a negative perception rather than opening up another way of seeing and being seen. This generated considerable discussion in the group about the potential dangers of making assumptions generally, as well as in relation to spirituality.

Many ways not one way

The sense of 'many ways not one way' outlined in postmodern thinking was reinforced by Monica's and Teresa's experience, where it was so clear that each of them found it difficult to accept the other's preferences. Most pairs of participants experienced differences. Even within a relatively small group, there was a considerable variety in how spirituality was expressed. Some people could see this as interesting or stimulating rather than challenging, but the implications for practice were clear to all. What was also clear was the need to let go of the binary of right/wrong. Several participants commented that, intellectually, they absolutely agreed their way wasn't *the* way, but that it was harder emotionally to agree there were other ways that were equally valid. There was consensus that this fitted with cultural pressure for there to be *the* answer. This connected to the following point.

Recognising the influence of social and personal context and history

Critical social theory affirms the importance of understanding the influence of culture and history in reflecting critically on practice. Daloz (2000: 113) suggests the value for transformative learning of 'conscious, critical reflection on our early assumptions about how life is'. In reacting to Monica and Teresa, several people in the group were able to make connections to their own history and social context: for one, growing up in a primarily Catholic small town and experiencing mutual support and inclusion within that community. Another linked her more negative attitudes to religion to seeing groups of children from different religious-based schools calling each other names.

This also led to a discussion about the influence of the social context and history in general: what in the culture affected perceptions of spirituality and religion? How had individuals internalised these ideas? Most of the participants had grown up in Australia, often described as a secular country, and could see how a primarily Christian culture continued to have an impact on social policies such as gay marriage, funding of private schools, attitudes to newly arrived Muslims, and spiritual practices of Indigenous people. This led to a discussion about how social context influences the experience of being different, which raised questions about fairness and social justice: how could practitioners influence the prevailing culture, organisationally and more generally, to be more inclusive. This led to the following point.

The challenge of actively valuing difference

This was particularly poignant, in this example, given that both participants were from similar backgrounds. While Monica acknowledged there were aspects of Catholicism she found challenging, another assumption for her was that it was better to stay and try to change it, given what worked. Teresa's assumption was that if you didn't like a particular form of spiritual expression, you should find another that suited you better, or create your own.

The group were fascinated as well as somewhat challenged by these and other differences and the potential conflicts they could see. What emerged was that, for many, it felt easier somehow to be respectful of someone operating from a completely different place – for example, a Baptist working with a Hindu – as they would have fewer built-in expectations. The past assumption had been that it would be easier to work with someone similar to oneself. This raised issues about how to actively accept and work with difference, to contribute to a more socially just way of operating; a questioning of making assumptions in general. It also generated discussion about how to actively value difference in practice – how to change community norms as well as organisational culture – as Modood (2008: 39) puts it, 'the right to have one's "difference" recognised and supported in both the public and the private sphere.'

Limits to expression of difference in spirituality

One of the potential tensions between a postmodern and critical social theory approach is the issue of the limits to valuing difference. This is a particularly confronting issue in practice: are there some activities or perspectives that should not be tolerated? How do you distinguish between what you are finding personally unacceptable and what would be professionally and socially unacceptable? Initially, for example, Monica questioned whether Wiccan practices would compromise Teresa's health and, if so, was it reasonable to refuse to support her with it? She later conceded that this related more to lack of knowledge about Wiccan ways, but the question remained in the group. Starting from a premise of socially just and inclusive practice helped, with an expectation that abusive practices were not acceptable.

Connecting reflection to action

Thinking about what they would want from a professional led participants to identify what needed to change in themselves: being aware of, and if necessary changing, their own assumptions, attitudes and values. A common desire was to be treated as a 'normal' whole person, not an illness. Some were conscious of how they didn't always manage this with their clients, and explored how a changed assumption might lead to changed behaviour. Monica's and Teresa's example generated discussion about developing the capacity to let go of assumptions and to ask about meaning rather than to assume knowledge. At an organisational level, participants could also see the need for change, in attitudes, rules, organisational assumptions and arrangements – from simply allowing conversations about what matters, to renaming the chapel as a centre for spirituality. While the thought of community change was daunting, several participants could see opportunities for at least having different kinds of conversations: naming spirituality rather than avoiding it.

Emerging assumptions regarding professional practice and practice within organisations

The assumptions that surfaced from this discussion were typical of those explored in workshops. The key assumptions, as individuals named them from this experience, were:

- spirituality is a significant aspect of how people live, and should be included in work with clients
- the whole person is important, including their spirituality
- my own spirituality has an impact on my work
- workers need to be open to clients' expressions of the spiritual and of what works for them
- difference should be celebrated, not just accepted
- workers need to recognise when their own spirituality is getting in the way of someone else's
- organisations need to recognise the importance of spirituality as part of practice and to build in support/supervision for workers.

Formal evaluations

Feedback from those who participated in the one day workshops suggested the value of exploring and reflecting on their personal experience of spirituality, as well as their reactions to situations involving spiritual issues for others. These fitted with the results from a more formal evaluation related to the set of workshops connected to the Pastoral Care Networks Project (Gardner and Nolan, 2009). Thirty of those who participated in the training were interviewed at least six months after training was completed. Participants were asked about what difference, if any, the training had made; what dilemmas or issues, if any, had emerged from using the training; and, in retrospect, what was useful about the training and anything they would have liked to be different.

The major differences for practice that emerged were:

- **Becoming more aware** – eleven felt they had an increased sense of recognising their own values, their own spirituality in the sense of meaning, and their own reactions, and so were more able to recognise how they might be unconsciously influencing others. Increased awareness was also an outcome for the Fook and Gardner (2007) participants. This connected to …

- **Being more open to difference** – eleven named this change, which nine said helped them to be more open or less rigid in their expectations of others: 'I have learnt about accepting people where they're at and I'm learning not to judge or become frustrated.' Fook and Gardner (2007) participants named this as 'new ways of seeing', which generated a greater sense of their capacity to act. This was consistent with the participants from the spirituality workshops, and many gave examples of such changed actions as …

- **Having different conversations, including spirituality** – eleven said they now had conversations that included spirituality, particularly for some having a greater depth of conversation: 'go deeper now', another 'allowing more time for reflection and relationship'. Similarly, Fook and Gardner's (2007: 133) participants expressed their desire to respond in a fuller, 'human, holistic way'.

- **Feeling more confident in relating to clients** – eight felt more comfortable in having 'these kinds of conversations' with clients; six specifically had shifted from feeling they had to have answers to being able 'just to sit and listen, which is what people want'. This was partly a greater comfort in sitting with uncertainty, not having to have the 'right' answer, and in tolerating ambiguity, also identified by Fook and Gardner (2007) participants.

- **Recognising their own spirituality** – six saw this as a significant change, and for some this connected to …

- **Increased care for self** – six were more conscious of taking care of themselves – at least so that they could care for others.

- **Developing and extending networks** – this related to sharing the experience of training. Six commented that the training had developed, extended and/or deepened their networks, with four feeling increased mutual support.

Again this fits with outcomes identified in Fook and Gardner (2007: 139) that critical reflection encourages a shared sense of experience and values.

Few dilemmas or issues were raised that participants felt unable to manage. However, there was a small group of three who commented on their organisation's lack of understanding of spirituality and the need to seek organisational change. This included their new assumptions: that spirituality should be part of all roles, not exclusively a specialist one. Reynolds and Vince (2004) advocate implementing critical reflection at an organisational level to achieve organisational change rather than expecting this to come only from changed individual practice.

Implications for using critical reflection and spirituality in professional training and practice

The centrality of experience

Reflecting on experience from this particular example contributed significantly to the power of this workshop for all participants. First, there was the experience of articulating what would be important for each participant if faced with serious illness or death – in itself a reflective activity that many described as challenging. Second, the experience of sharing in pairs and being – in some cases, at least – confronted with the differences between self and other. Third, the experience of exploring this in the group generated reflection, including seeing how different experiences of 'spirituality' can be. Providing some experiences that could be considered spiritual, such as a meditation, offered another form of experience, which again demonstrated that people react differently. Working with experience included recognising and validating participants' emotional responses as useful forms of knowledge.

The value of working in groups

This example reinforces the value of working in groups for critical reflection and for training in spirituality. Hearing from others about their different assumptions is much more powerful than being told about them. In a group, participants hear and react to a wider range of examples and reactions. Some commented that hearing about someone else's experience that connected to theirs allowed them to gain a new perspective on it.

The need to articulate underlying assumptions and values of individuals and organisations

Enabling individuals to name underlying assumptions and values meant participants could quickly see that they were coming from different perspectives. Making the assumptions explicit clarified both where there were differences, and also where there was common ground, particularly in shared underlying values.

The need for understanding and change

The exercises demonstrated participants' need both to understand their own attitudes and values in relation to spirituality, and to be able to determine how to change these to practise in spiritually sensitive ways.

Impact on organisations and practice

Feedback from this and other workshops affirms that spirituality is increasingly seen as an essential part of practice in health and social care organisations. Participants indicated that after training they saw their practice more holistically, which they felt would make their practice more rewarding for both them and their clients. Many felt more aware of their own assumptions and values and the potential impact of this on practice. Some identified operating differently: having conversations that include spirituality, being able to value 'being with' clients as much as doing.

Having recognised for themselves their capacity to work holistically, including the spiritual in practice, participants wanted this acknowledged by their organisation. For many organisations, this role was seen as belonging to a pastoral care worker or chaplain, and participants now felt it should be part of everyone's role – given training and interest. The role of the chaplain could then be as a supportive specialist, available for support and consultation for staff as well as referral for more complex spiritual issues. Given the limited time chaplains had, this made sense to participants, though not necessarily to their organisations or to chaplains themselves. Participants also identified a need for continuing training, support and supervision or consultation. In one organisation, staff started a mutually supportive supervision group, meeting monthly and using exercises of the type used in training.

Future implications

The experience used here suggests the value of integrating critical reflection and spirituality or developing 'critical spirituality'. Critical reflection and spirituality can complement and strengthen each other, providing a holistic framework for practice. Including spirituality in practice clearly has value to practitioners, affirming the importance of what really matters that transcends the immediate. The spiritual, meditative or contemplative way of being can encourage the capacity to sit with uncertainty and not knowing. Many clients desire the inclusion of spirituality in how they are perceived and engaged with by professionals. For those who participated in workshops, identifying spirituality broadly and inclusively was helpful in reminding them of what this meant for themselves and others, as well as acknowledging difference.

At least some aspects of religious and spiritual traditions advocate for more socially just and inclusive ways, and contribute knowledge about how to do this.

At the same time, it is clear that working with spirituality is often profoundly challenging to professionals' own assumptions and values, which can be so deeply embedded that they are difficult to identify. Critical reflection processes enable feelings, thoughts, assumptions and values to be articulated and constructively affirmed and/or confronted in a culture of acceptance. The theories underlying critical reflection help this: reflexivity illustrates the complexity of perceptions; reflective practice reminds practitioners to check whether their espoused theory fits how they act in practice; postmodernism and critical social theory encourage explorations of how social and personal history has influenced assumptions and values, and of possibilities for change.

Combining critical reflection with spirituality then affirms working in a holistic way, valuing difference and appreciating the influences of personal and social history and context.

Critical spirituality acknowledges that there are times when the dilemmas of difference need to be named and accepted or connected with, rather than expecting agreement or resolution. What is more important is the willingness to engage in respectful and active discussion with clearly non-violent boundaries, and the capacity to manage uncertainty. The 'critical' in critical reflection can engage with the liberation theology aspects of religious traditions to reinforce the influence of social context for individuals and communities, and to make explicit the value of a socially just and actively inclusive approach.

There are clearly implications for organisations in taking seriously the inclusion of a critical spirituality approach to practice. Practitioners will need training, continuing support, and a combination of accessible consultation and/or supervision. Those providing this will also need training in critical spirituality practices. More challenging for organisations may be the implication that taking seriously a critical spirituality approach means being willing to seek change at organisational, community and social levels, as well as with individuals and families.

References

Abbas, S.Q. and Panjwani, S. (2008) 'The necessity of spiritual care towards the end of life', *Ethics and Medicine*, 24(2): 113–18.

Banks, S. (2008) 'Critical commentary: social work ethics', *British Journal of Social Work*, 38: 1238–49.

——(2010) 'Integrity in professional life: issues of conduct, commitment and capacity', *British Journal of Social Work*, 40: 2168–84.

Berry, T. (2009) *The Christian Future and the Fate of Earth*, NY: Orbis Books.

Canda, E.R. and Furman, L.D. (2010) *Spiritual Diversity in Social Work Practice: The Heart of Helping* (2nd edn), Oxford: Oxford University Press.

Daloz, L.A.P. (2000) 'Transformative learning for the common good', in Mezirow, J. (ed.), *Learning as Transformation*, San Francisco: Jossey-Bass.

Fook, J. and Gardner, F. (2007) *Practising Critical Reflection: A Resource Handbook*, Maidenhead: Open University Press.

Fook, J., Ryan, M.A. and Hawkins, L. (2000) *Professional Expertise: Practice, Theory and Education for Working in Uncertainty*, London: Whiting & Birch.

Fook, J., White, S.A. and Gardner, F. (2006) 'Critical reflection: a review of contemporary literature and understandings', in White, S., Fook, J. and Gardner, F. (eds), *Critical Reflection and Professional Practice*, London: Open University Press.

Forman, R. (2004) *Grassroots Spirituality*, Exeter: Imprint Academic.

Fowler, J.W. (1981) *Stages of Faith: The Psychology of Human Development and the Quest for Meaning*, San Francisco: Harper & Row.

Gardner, F. (2011) *Critical Spirituality: A Holistic Approach to Contemporary Practice*, Farnham: Ashgate.

Gardner, F. and Nolan, I. (2009) *Pastoral Care Works Project Final Evaluation*, Melbourne: Palliative Care Unit, La Trobe University.

Gilligan, P. (2009) 'Considering religion and beliefs in child protection and safeguarding work: is any consensus emerging?', *Child Abuse Review*, 18(2): 94–110.

Gray, M. and Lovat, T. (2008) 'Practical mysticism, Habermas, and social work praxis', *Journal of Social Work*, 8(2): 149–62.

Gross, R.M. (2009) *A Garland of Feminist Reflections: Forty Years of Religious Exploration*, Berkeley, CA: University of California.

Gustafsson, G., Eriksson, S., Strandberg, G. and Norberg, A. (2010) 'Burnout and perceptions of conscience among health care personnel: a pilot study', *Nursing Ethics*, 17(1): 23–38.

al-Haqq Kugle, S.S. (2010) *Homosexuality in Islam: Critical Reflection on Gay, Lesbian and Transgender Muslims*, Oxford: Oneworld Publications.

Haynes, A., Hilbers, J., Kivikko, J. and Ratnatvyuha (2007) *Spirituality and Religion in Health Care Practice: A Person-Centred Resource for Staff at the Prince of Wales Hospital, Sydney*, Sydney: South Eastern Sydney Illawarra Area Health Service.

Heelas, P.A. and Woodhead, L. (2005) *The Spiritual Revolution: Why Religion is Giving Way to Spirituality*, Oxford: Blackwell Publishing.

Helmeke, K.B. and Sori, C.F. (eds) (2006) *The Therapist's Notebook for Integrating Spirituality in Counselling*, Binghampton, NY: Haworth Press.

Hodge, D. (2011) 'Using spiritual interventions in practice: developing some guidelines from evidence-based practice', *Social Work*, 56(2): 149–58.

Hoffman, L., Cox, R.H., Ervin-Cox, B. and Mitchell, M. (2005) 'Training issues in spirituality and psychotherapy: a foundational approach', in Cox, R.H., Ervin-Cox, B. and Hoffman, L. (eds), *Spirituality and Psychological Health*, Colorado Springs, CO: Colorado School of Professional Psychology Press, 3–14.

Holloway, M.A. and Moss, B. (2010) *Spirituality and Social Work*, Houndmills: Palgrave Macmillan.

Johns, C. (2005) 'Balancing the winds', *Reflective Practice*, 6(1): 67–84.

Kamitsuka, M.D. (2007) *Feminist Theology and the Challenge of Difference*, Oxford: Oxford University Press.

Kavanagh, J. (2007) *The World is our Cloister, A Guide to the Modern Religious Life*, Winchester: O Books, John Hunt Publishing.

Laabs, C. (2011) 'Perceptions of moral integrity: contradictions in need of explanation', *Nursing Ethics*, 18(3): 431–40.

Lartey, E.Y. (2003) *In Living Color: An Intercultural Approach to Pastoral Care and Counseling*, London and Philadelphia: Jessica Kingsley.

MacKinlay, E. (2008) 'Perspective on the development of knowledge of spirituality and aging in nursing and pastoral care: an Australian context', *Journal of Religion, Spirituality and Aging*, 20(1/2): 135–52.

Martin, S. (2009) 'Illness of the mind or illness of the spirit? Mental health-related conceptualization and practices of older Iranian immigrants', *Health & Social Work*, 34(2): 117–26.

McCurdy, D. (2008) 'Ethical spiritual care at the end of life', *American Journal of Nursing*, 108(5): 11–12.

McSherry, W. (2007) *The Meaning of Spirituality and Spiritual Care within Nursing and Health Care Practice*, London: Quay Books.

Modood, T. (2008) 'Muslims, equality and secularism', in Spalek, B. and Imtoual, A. (eds), *Religion, Spirituality and the Social Sciences: Challenging Marginalisation*, Bristol: Bristol University Press, 37–49.

Murray, J.S. (2010) 'Moral courage in healthcare: acting ethically even in the presence of risk', *Online Journal of Issues in Nursing*, 15(3): 16–25.

Ní Raghallaigh, M. (2011) 'Religion in the lives of unaccompanied minors: an available and compelling coping resource', *British Journal of Social Work*, 41(3): 539–56.

Nichols, L. and Hunt, B. (2011) 'The significance of spirituality for individuals with chronic illness: implications for mental health counseling', *Journal of Mental Health Counseling*, 33(1): 51–65.

Reynolds, M.A. and Vince, R. (eds) (2004) *Organizing Reflection*, Aldershot: Ashgate.

Rowland, C. (ed.) (1999) *The Cambridge Companion to Liberation Theology*, Cambridge: Cambridge University Press.

Ruether, R. (1985) *Womanguides: Readings Towards a Feminist Theology*, Boston, MA: Beacon Press.

——(2006) *Goddesses and the Divine Feminine: A Western Religious History*, Berkeley, CA: University of California Press.

Rumbold, B. (ed.) (2002). *Spirituality and Palliative Care*, Melbourne: Oxford University Press.

Schön, D.A. (1983) *The Reflective Practitioner: How Professionals Think in Action*, New York: Basic Books.

Sneed, R.A. (2010) *Representations of Homosexuality: Black Liberation Theology and Cultural Criticism*, New York: Palgrave Macmillan.

Stirling, B., Furman, L.D., Benson, P.W., Canda, E.R. and Grimwood, C. (2010) 'A comparative survey of Aotearoa New Zealand and UK social workers on the role of religion and spirituality in practice', *British Journal of Social Work*, 40(2): 602–21.

Swinton, J. (2001) *Spirituality and Mental Health Care*, London: Jessica Kingsley.

Trelfa, J. (2005) 'Faith in reflective practice', *Reflective Practice*, 6(2): 205–12.

Vernon, M. (2007). *After Atheism: Science, Religion and the Meaning of Life*, Houndmills: Palgrave Macmillan.

White, G. (2006) *Talking about Spirituality in Health Care Practice*, London: Jessica Kingsley.

Wilber, K. (1997) *The Eye of Spirit*, Boston: Shambhala.

Winslow, G.R. and Wehtje-Winslow, B. (2007) 'Ethical boundaries of spiritual care', *Medical Journal of Australia*, 186(10): S63–S66.

Wong, Y.-L.R. and Vinsky, J. (2009) 'Speaking from the margins: a critical reflection on the "spiritual-but-not-religious" discourse in social work', *British Journal of Social Work*, 39(7): 1343–59.

4 Not beating around the bush

Critical reflection in a rural community health service

Gavan Thomson[1,2]

This is an account of the first six years of critical reflection, from early 2005 until mid-2011, enjoyed by a group of community development and health promotion practitioners at a rural community health service. The author was a founding member of the group, and remains in it.

The place

Cobaw Community Health is located in the Macedon Ranges Shire in Victoria, Australia, a rural shire with a population of about 40,000, with no town of more than 12,000 inhabitants. Cobaw sits in a unique sector of the health and welfare industry in Australia, namely the independent community health sector, which exists only in the state of Victoria. It was established in the mid-1970s by the progressive federal Labor government, although health remains mainly the responsibility of state governments. Victorian state governments have differed greatly in their support for the sector and many of the reforming objectives of the community health movement have been lost, but the sector survives as a strong advocate for the health needs of less advantaged community members. Forty independent community health services continue, each an independent legal entity.

Cobaw provides a broad range of health and welfare services, with an annual budget of approximately $4.5 million and about eighty-five full- and part-time staff. Most funding comes from state government through many program streams; other money is from federal government, philanthropic grants, fees and donations. Its catchment ranges from the metropolitan fringe growth corridors, across traditional farming and equine land, to pockets of real social disadvantage, isolation and rural poverty.

Cobaw's services fit three broad categories: direct service such as allied health and counselling, youth work and housing support; health promotion (HP), which includes adult day activity and family day care for children, and a range of activity and support groups; and community development (CD) projects, with broader developmental objectives. CD has consisted of the Way Out project (addressing homophobia and supporting same-sex-attracted young people across rural Victoria); the School Focused Youth Service (supporting the mental wellbeing of young people across three shires); the Community Garden Project established on Cobaw's land; Youthinc, an underage alcohol diversion program; L2P, a learner-driver mentoring program; Parent Buddies, a family strengthening and support project; and the Macedon Ranges VCAL, an education course re-engaging young people.

Cobaw has a contemporary corporate structure, with staff in teams under team coordinators who sit under a senior program manager, who reports to the Chief Executive Officer. A local Board of Directors employs the CEO and sets the strategic and policy framework. Teams are based upon foci of work, except for a number of CD and HP workers, who instead report directly to a senior manager. Some of these workers have the status of coordinators, while most do not. These workers formed the critical reflection group described here.

Starting the group

In 2004, Cobaw introduced a new level of management, appointing two senior managers. One was keen to introduce group supervision for the teams under her. A social worker, she became aware of the Critical Reflection approach then being developed by Jan Fook and Fiona Gardner (2002) at the Centre for Professional Development, La Trobe University in the regional city of Bendigo. Links between Cobaw and social work on this campus have been strong, with a number of the social workers employed at Cobaw having trained there. The approach was first adopted by the counselling team at Cobaw after Jan Fook conducted training. Afterwards, discussions took place between myself and the manager about the supervision needs of the CD and HP workers outside teams, and she formed a group for us, using this critical reflection approach. Training for group members was conducted in 2004 by Fiona Gardner, after which formal critical reflection for the group commenced, and has continued since on a monthly basis, with Fiona as our facilitator.

When the group started, the manager, the group members and the facilitator agreed on two main aims:

- to form a group where people trusted each other sufficiently to debrief, and to explore more deeply work-related experiences that were frustrating or troubling in some way
- to use those experiences to develop the group's 'theory of practice' about CD and HP in the agency.

The expectation was that sharing about practice would lead to common understandings of good practice, which the group would then promote within the agency as its preferred approach to CD and HP.

Membership of the group has been fluid. In all, twelve workers have passed through the group, while four have stayed from the beginning to the time of writing, the author included. This reflects the turnover in workers and programs in the CD and HP sectors. Orientating new members has been for-malised twice, when Fiona presented a brief theory and practice 'refresher' when a number of new members had joined. Otherwise, new members have been briefed and have become acculturated through observing and participating.

The list of positions and roles of members shows the group's diversity:

- Family Strengthening project officer
- Health Promotion coordinator
- School Focused Youth Service coordinator (the author)
- L2P project officer (volunteer mentoring of youth learner drivers)
- WayOut project coordinator
- WayOut project worker
- Parenting Buddies worker
- Youthinc project officers (two) (under-age alcohol diversion)
- Community Garden project officer
- Planned Activity Group coordinators (two).

A range of professionals have been members of the group, including four social workers, plus dietitian, registered nurse, health promoter, public health, disability, youth worker, and family support.

The group at work

The group has followed the model of critical reflection developed by Fook and Gardner (2002). At the beginning, the group was very keen to negotiate comprehensive ground rules, which have remained ever since. While the need for such rules was raised in training (Fook and Gardner, 2007), it was of particular concern to our group that the rules were adequate and explicit. The most important relate to privacy and confidentiality. The first is that the proceedings of sessions were not to be reported, or available, to the man-agement of the agency, although a worker has sole discretion about whether to take their reflections to their supervising manager or team leader. The second relates to confidentiality of sessions, and involves disclosing nothing about the content of sessions unless it is completely de-identified. The third is about members' safety. We agreed that outside of sessions, we are not to refer to any issue presented by a member unless that member raises the issue first. This has been called 'not referring to others' material', and seeks to ensure that a member controls any raising of their own 'problems, failings or inadequacies'. Over the life of the group, there has been no occasion when anyone has raised a concern about breaches of ground rules. Often we have had a worker and their supervisor in the group, which has been acknowl-edged on occasion, and appears to work fine in that no member of the group has articulated that this has affected their choice or content of incident. Noble and Irwin (2009: 355) suggest that a critical reflection group is more likely to be aware of issues of power, and that critical reflection has the potential to 'democratize the process'. The positive experience of the 'supervisees' might support this, and indicate that our processes have resulted in 'power to' rather than 'power over'.

The group generally meets monthly (usually eleven times per annum) and almost always for two hours. Each session is made up of three possible foci: at stage one, a worker presenting a critical incident; and a member's stage two from the previous meeting being examined, or the group working on an issue in common to do with work within the agency. In general, the consideration of a critical incident (either at stage one or stage two) takes up one hour, half the session. The sessions mix and match these different foci, depending on the needs of the group. Sometimes two stage ones would be presented in a session; other times, two stage twos; otherwise a stage one and a stage two, etc. Over the years, all possible combinations have eventuated.

There is no roster for when a member presents, or even an expectation that a member 'should', beyond a general awareness that it is not good to 'hog' the sessions if someone who has not had a go for a while is keen. Although there is no agreement that a new member must present, it is generally assumed that they will eventually, and this has been the case. No record is kept of who has presented when, and this means that some members clearly present more than others, but no-one has minded. A critical incident is whatever a group member wants it to be (the only constraint being that it must be about work). Incidents have included issues of immediate concern, patterns over time, and incidents from the past that are not fully resolved, such as conflicts, complaints made against a worker, frustrations about support, role clarity and resources, difficulties in working with other individuals, organisations or sectors, relationships with management, work-related depression and anxiety, program constraints, and lack of clarity in roles and resources.

Stages one and two

Presenting a critical incident has remained a formal process. When it is agreed who is to present a stage one, that member comes with a written summary of their incident under three headings: background to the incident; the incident; and how the incident has affected me. Copies are distributed, then collected at the end. These summaries have varied between 150 and 500 words, and are used as a discussion starter. They also serve the critical purpose of affording the opportunity to reflect before the session and to organise the incident into a framework that focuses on personal impact. Stage one involves the worker presenting the incident, clarifying anything that is not clear, and then brainstorming, with input from all present, the context to the incident, both broad and narrow. The possible assumptions of other people involved (and not present) can also be brainstormed, explored and captured. The session then focuses on uncovering, clarifying and recording what assumptions the worker makes that relate to the incident, and what values and beliefs might underpin these assumptions. The facilitator takes notes, ideally on a copying whiteboard. Problem-solving, developing strategies, solution-creating and other attempts to address the impact of the incident, or to stop it recurring, are deliberately eschewed here. (This can be a challenge for new members and 'task-focused' members.) In preparation for stage two, the presenter takes with them the notes made, capturing the context and the assumptions.

The second session starts with a brief summary of the incident, followed by an update on any related developments since the first session. Then the assumptions that were recorded in the first session are systematically worked through with the presenter. The presenter is encouraged and prompted to reflect on each assumption and relate any new realisation, thinking or behaviour that may have occurred since the first session. Often the worker will not want to alter an assumption or belief, but reaffirm this instead. Again, these are written up for the presenter to take away. The worker is encouraged to describe any changes they may want to implement as a result of the reflection; and finally, the worker is given the opportunity to come up with a slogan or catch-cry that captures their new understanding.

An example

Below is a critical incident presented by the author some six years ago. It was chosen from the thirteen critical incidents I have presented over the years, at an average of two per year.

Critical incident

Background

My program, the School Focused Youth Service (SFYS), aims to improve the system for meeting the support and intervention needs of young people aged ten to eighteen years who are at risk of suicide or self-harm. The SFYS seeks to build collaboration, partnerships, supports and links between the education sector and the health, welfare and youth sectors. It was established following the Victorian Suicide Prevention Taskforce (Kirby) report in the late 1990s, which found that 'silos' existed between the sectors, making collaboration and system-building difficult. As a sole worker across three rural local government areas, I have sixty schools to service from the three different educations sectors: state, Catholic and independent. And I seek to support, resource, fund and organise with, between and within these schools to achieve the aims of the program. I came to this position as a social worker with no experience of the secondary school education sector since I left high school three decades ago. As a program that no school has any obligation to engage with, the SFYS has no mandate for school involvement.

The incident

As I am based in a community health centre, I am outside the education silo. I experience the same barriers in seeking access to schools that the SFYS was set up to address. I often feel that I am an outsider from the education sector. There are schools I know I can support that will not engage with me. Even the student welfare staff in the schools seem reluctant to engage with me. I find it much easier to work with the other (non-education) sectors, where I am welcomed readily, yet this is not my primary focus. The student wellbeing unit and workers within the Department of Education, which partly funds the program, seem intent, in my view, on keeping the SFYS out.

How the incident has affected me

I feel anxious and frustrated by the need constantly to promote myself and my service to many schools, often with little effect. I feel like an outsider who is not welcome in schools and not able to be of any benefit to schools. It feels like I am bashing my head against a brick wall. There must be a better way to practise social work.

From this presentation, the stage one critical reflection session generated a number of my assumptions and beliefs about the incident. These were written up on a copying whiteboard, and I left the session with the copy.

The most relevant assumptions are summarised as follows.

Stage one: key assumptions

In this role, being an outsider is bad while being an insider is good.
It's hard to be an outsider.
It would be so much easier if I was working inside the education sector.
I must get all schools on side and accessed.
Those I cannot access really need my service, in fact there is a direct inverse relationship between access and need.
Persistence will triumph in the end so I just have to persist.

Workers in the education sector are somehow different, and resistant to a better system

One month later, we undertook stage two. With the usual hurly burly of work life, I had not deliberately set aside time to reflect on the incident, but many times it had popped into my head. From the start of the second session, it became clear to me (and the group) that my thinking about the incident was very black-and-white, and that 'false dichotomies' of good and bad have pervaded my assumptions. Below is a summary of the stage two report highlighting how I had reflected on each assumption.

Stage two: assumptions reconsidered

In this role, being an outsider is bad while being an insider is good

This is a false dichotomy – there is a gradation between 'insideness' and 'outsideness'. And there are clear disadvantages in being an insider, and clear advantages in being an outsider to the education sector. These include not being under the policy or procedural constraints in the education sector; having the ability to be a dispassionate supporter in all schools; not being bound to a particular educational sector, school or bureaucracy; and not being co-opted or ordered to respond to individual student welfare crises or case work in schools.

It's hard to be an outsider

The system can clearly be changed from without, and I have been able to find some allies and support in the education sector where I have been welcomed and where I have been able to contribute. I am an insider to my program and my agency, where I best 'belong'. In these settings I have the 'power' and constraints of an insider. Any work across sectors will necessitate being both an insider and an outsider.

It would be so much easier if I was working inside the education sector

From the above, there would be clear disadvantages to working inside the sector, which might well make the job harder, not easier. Being mandated may make the role harder because meaningful cooperation and partnership can only come out of interest and consent, while educators entering into unwilling connection with me would create a whole new problem.

I must get all schools on side and accessed

'Sometimes a horse will even refuse to be led to water.' School leadership and staff may not cooperate for a variety of reasons. Systemic change can be slow and involves the innovators changing first. There is no point devoting too many resources to areas where access is proving to be impossible. However, open communication with all schools is important. The catchment area and the number of schools are too great anyway, which would make it impossible to work with all schools.

Those I cannot access really need my service, in fact there is a direct inverse relationship between access and need

This is a false assumption. Schools that do not access me may not need my services. My program is not the only pathway for a school to provide excellence in student wellbeing. Needs change in schools from time to time, and are more to do with school leadership, personnel, culture and circumstances than connection with me.

Persistence will triumph in the end so I just have to persist

There is a limit to how far persistence will go. Persisting with what does not work is futile. Trying new ways, being flexible and staying available are as important. There are instances when I have been contacted 'out of the blue' by school leaders who were well aware of my service, but had not used it before. This demonstrates the importance of awareness, communication and availability.

Workers in the education sector are somehow different, and resistant to a better system

As in all large and diverse sectors, there will be a continuum of workers' values and beliefs. The challenge is to engage those who support the aims of my program, and to offer something that has meaning for them.

At the end of this session, I was able to sum up with the semi-serious slogan that I would be the 'Welcome Stranger' – an 'outsider' who is welcomed into schools and brings 'golden' opportunities. (This is a reference to a famous, massive gold nugget found locally in the nineteenth century called the Welcome Stranger – for obvious reasons.) Some years on, I often bring this slogan to mind when I front the reception at a school and sign the visitors' book, and it continues to help.

Common themes

Approximately 100 critical incidents have been raised in the group over the years. Common themes have arisen, which are almost always about the tensions workers face in attempting to do good CD and HP practice within contexts familiar to most of the group members. Themes resonate frequently with group members, such that a sense of 'my incidents are your incidents' has arisen. Such themes often relate to broader social structures and power, as Brookfield (2005) outlined, and can be organised under the four headings below.

Preferred practice approach by the worker being compromised

Example: a group member struggles with addressing problems and conflict in a project in the agency. The worker is concerned that, although the project has obvious CD objectives, there is no clear CD approach or plan in place, and few resources.

Tension caused by the dominant focus and culture within the organisation, and the internal relationships that result

Example: a group member feels that their program is relatively under-resourced after the allocation of program budgets within the agency.

Limitations in the parameters placed around the group member's programs and projects – agency , partnership or funders' parameters

Example: a worker struggles with facilitating sector networks after the regional office of the relevant government department withdraws funding and other resourcing from these networks.

General dilemmas of community work – dealing with injustices, domination, power and influence in the groups and people with which members work

Example: a group member organises and runs a network with a counterpart from a different organisation. However, the worker experiences the partner as domineering, insensitive, uncooperative and disrespectful of others.

The second aim – towards a theory of practice

Our aim of developing a theory of practice for CD and HP work within the agency is different from the usual approaches to supervision or reflection. Critical reflection leads us to examine our individual assumptions and allows us to affirm or change these assumptions. Importantly, it also gives us the capacity to reflect collectively on the assumptions associated with our organisation's way of operating. The capacity of the group to spend time focusing on common issues and develop common theories and strategies was built in from the start as the means of addressing the second aim of the group. It has remained a feature of the group, and complements well the individual critical incident reflections. We have generated change at both individual and organisational levels. This emphasis away from the individual has been a group feature and meets the challenge of Reynolds and Vince (2004), who critiqued critical reflection for an overemphasis on individual reflection. Time devoted to addressing common issues would probably have taken up 25–30% of the sessions. At times, this focus has dominated group proceedings, while in other periods it has not arisen. The group has used this time, by and large, to consider the two complementary questions of how to strengthen our position within the organisation, and how to respond to organisational issues that affect us.

Embedding community development and health promotion

One major group involvement has been in the agency's strategic planning, and this has resulted in documenting and presenting good practice for the agency in a number of forums. During the development of Cobaw's 2007 strategic plan, the group deliberately sought to advocate for strengthening the commitment to CD and HP approaches at an overarching level. This arose from a shared understanding that, although the agency has made a firm commitment to the social model of health, which includes key CD and HP concepts, in practice the strategic commitment to CD and HP work could be improved. The group agreed that the implementation of these approaches remained limited and poorly understood across programs.

The group presented a full day's workshop for members of the strategic planning group, comprising board members and senior staff. The workshop was facilitated by three members of the group, and led to Cobaw including in its strategic plan as a priority 'the embedding of health promotion and community development across the organisation'. The teams' annual planning template was modified to include CD and HP activities, and all teams were asked to include these in their plans.

In 2009, Cobaw management invited group members to conduct a review of these components in team plans. Group members interviewed teams about this work and analysed this section of all team plans. Many staff reported a limited understanding of, and little experience with, CD and HP approaches, while some team plans had not included what could be considered as core HP or CD work. Based on these findings, members of the group were then engaged to conduct two half-day in-house workshops for all Cobaw staff: one on HP and one on CD. Following these workshops, many ideas were generated by teams for CD and HP projects, and our group members offered to assist and support teams in planning or undertaking such work.

At each stage of these involvements in the strategic planning and direction of the organisation, the group has been able to reflect powerfully on the next strategic step. This has resulted in acquiring some wisdom about sustainability and progress in the context where the group is at the margin of a larger organisation focused necessarily on dealing with thousands of individual clients.

Developing shared understandings, strategies and action

Other instances of adopting a common strategy include the following:

- A perceived lack of clarity around performance and dismissal processes raised concern for some group members. After reflection, the group was able to participate in negotiating, drafting and implementing new employee performance, appraisal and disciplinary policies in the organisation.
- A community garden project established by Cobaw on its land was experiencing considerable difficulties, which affected a number of group members. The group was able to develop an evaluation and restructuring strategy, which the agency adopted as a way forward.
- As is the case in many rural agencies, access to work cars had become a source of tension for some group members who travelled long distances during and outside business hours. The group submitted a paper to

management outlining issues and making recommendations. This contributed to a review of car use, and to new guidelines being adopted.

The group, over time, has developed a number of shared understandings of CD and HP practice. These regularly appear as motifs in the re-evaluation we undertake of our assumptions from stage one. The five key understandings are summarised below.

Collegial space

Many of the members of the group are sole workers in discrete areas of work; for us, the group offers a unique collegial space of great value. In the group, we can take the time to set aside tasks and share with our peers our often common concerns and dilemmas in a non-judgemental, informed, honest and open forum. The importance of this in sustaining effort and ensuring good practice in CD and HP work is hard to overemphasise.

Use of self

This concept has been front and centre in every session. It comprises the essence of reflexivity: understanding how I am perceived by others, how others respond to me, and how I perceive myself working with others. It also concerns how I think and feel about my work, how I perceive myself in the job, and what the job means to me. We often develop assumptions that we could or should do more, and that it is our own individual effort, skills, charisma and persistence that determine work success. Such assumptions about ourselves can mean we overlook the other micro- and macro-factors that have an impact on our job satisfaction and achievements, and on the CD and HP outcomes. These factors include resources, workload, access, opportunity, seniority and culture. When we bring these into our reflections, we get a more profound perception of ourselves at work and a more realistic understanding of what we do and don't bring. The feelings we have about our critical incidents seem, as Swan and Bailey (2004: 112) recognise, to be generated by the process itself. We have developed the ability to value strong feelings and to sit with a member who is crying or raging about their lot.

Funding and other resources

Not surprisingly, resourcing is a recurrent theme. Although each team member works in a separate program funding context, common understandings about funding have developed. Three considerations illustrate this: there is limited funding for CD and HP work in the sector; much of the available funding from philanthropic or government sources is of limited duration, usually one to three years; and the organisation has had a limited capacity to generate funds specifically for CD and HP. Thus, for CD and HP to be sustained, let alone prosper, we have reached the understanding that looking for and applying for funding is a central work role. Considerable expertise, experience and success in fund raising have been developed by group members as a result.

At home in the agency

The group clearly identifies with the overall goals of the organisation, and has no issue with the need for clinical services within a social model of health, but the predominance of these services in the agency creates tension. What it means to work in an organisation where the professional values we hold, the theories we adopt and the work we do are different from those of the majority in the organisation underlies some sessions. For example, the common data system is designed primarily to record individual client information and notes on one-to-one sessions. Members of our group had to enter their group's work in the database as a rolling series of 'anonymous events'. These circumstances affect our sense of belonging, connection, status and acceptance. And, more practically, they affect how we are managed and resourced, where we sit, literally and structurally, how we report, and how we are involved in the life of the agency. Some of our important actions as a group can be seen as attempts to nudge the core closer to us.

Slow work

Related to the differences above is the question of time. Group members appreciate that sustained change takes time: on one hand, there is no 'quick fix' in our work (though sometimes we look for it); on the other, there are broad countervailing forces that can undermine our work (but often we can't see these). The beauty of CR is that it provides some small antidote to the incessant tasks. In stage two, we have often come to understand how non-action and strategic retreat can be effective uses of time. We have also learnt to share strategies to deal with the economic rationalists' preference for tasks, not reflection; for action, not patience; for quantity, not quality; for interventions, not relationships; and for beans, not compost.

Future directions – dilemmas and opportunities

We have been going for quite a while, and as we come and go, dilemmas for the group recur. How do we best incorporate new members, and need they be doing similar work to us? If we stop having enough members for a group, and have to form a more heterogeneous group, will we lose our ability to reflect and act collectively? We are not an agency team, whereas all the other staff members are in teams. What are the pros and cons of being out of a team?

Another unresolved question is whether to encourage the agency to translate the shared learning from our critical reflection into agency policy and procedures. The agency has policy and procedures for much of its work, but not for our work practice. Would policy and procedures about the do's and don'ts of good practice in CD and HP help, hinder, or have no effect on the agency's continuing ability to maintain strong and successful CD and HP components with good staff?

One outgrowth has been the author becoming a critical reflection facilitator. I identified the need for group supervision for undersupported workers across my catchment, and for the past two years I have facilitated critical reflection groups. Being part of a critical reflection group at work has been of great benefit to me when on the other end of the whiteboard marker.

We have never formally evaluated our critical reflection group – which is surprising, upon reflection. But every so often, we have stopped to ask how it is going and whether we should continue. Yes has been our solid response.

Notes

1 Acknowledgement: I thank all my co-group members group over the years for their forbearance and assistance, and especially Julie Cairns, Kat Ettwell, Sue Hackney and Alicia O'Brien, the long-standing members, for providing feedback on this chapter. I also acknowledge the generosity of the senior managers at Cobaw Community Health, Anne McLennan, Gary Steadman and Margaret McDonald, who continue to support and resource critical reflection. I also thank my manager Gary Steadman for his feedback on this chapter.
2 Disclaimer: the views, opinions and interpretations expressed in this chapter are solely the author's and do not necessarily represent those of Cobaw Community Health.

References

Brookfield, S. (2005) *The Power of Critical Theory: Liberating Adult Learning and Teaching*, San Francisco: Jossey-Bass.

Fook, J. and Gardner, F. (2002) *Critical Reflection: Training Notes*. Bendigo: Centre for Professional Development, La Trobe University.

——(2007) *Practising Critical Reflection: A Resource Handbook*, Maidenhead: Open University Press.

Noble, C. and Irwin, J. (2009) 'Social work supervision: an exploration of the current challenges in a rapidly changing social, economic, and political environment', *Journal of Social Work*, 9(3): 345–58.

Reynolds, M. and Vince, R. (2004) 'Organizing reflection: an introduction', in Reynolds, M. and Vince, R. (eds), *Organizing Reflection*, Aldershot: Ashgate, 1–14.

Swan, E. and Bailey, A. (2004) 'Thinking with feeling: the emotions of reflection', in Reynolds, M. and Vince, R. (eds), *Organizing Reflection*, Aldershot: Ashgate, 105–25.

5 Learning critical reflection for professional practice

Helen Hickson

Starting to use critical reflection can be like finding yourself in the middle of a dark forest, surrounded by well-trodden paths. You see lots of paths and you have many options about which path to take, but that, in itself, can feel overwhelming. When you are learning the process of critical reflection you might feel lost, and you don't know where the paths will go – they are the paths that others have trodden. You might see a map of these paths, but it is important to find your own way and make your own map. At the start, it is scary to walk along a path not knowing where you might end up and what you might encounter along the way. As you develop a couple of well-trodden paths of your own, you begin to feel comfortable and you think that you can find your way out. But somehow, you always seem to find yourself back in the same place, in the middle of the dark forest. As you feel more confident, you are more willing to take a risk and explore what is beyond the path. You know the paths well enough to know that soon you will recognise a landmark or come across another well-trodden path, and you will know where you are, where you have come from and where you are going.

Introduction

I was drawn to critical reflection through my curiosity about ways to advance my skills in reflection and reflective practice. I enrolled in a short course in critical reflection, then a Master's program at La Trobe University in Bendigo, Australia, and I now find myself fascinated with critical reflection. I have developed a personal, professional and academic interest in critical reflection as I have pursued postgraduate study in this area. My PhD research explores the ways in which social workers learn, teach and use critical reflection.

There is a body of literature in which authors suggest that being reflective is essential in the contemporary workforce (Redmond, 2006; Fook and Gardner, 2007), yet little is understood about how people learn to be reflective and why people are drawn to reflective practice. Reflective practice literature is broad and influenced by many disciplines, and is therefore not confined to an approach used by social workers. While writers agree that there is value in reflective practice, definitions of terms such as reflection, critical reflection and reflective practice are contested, and writers from various disciplines use a range of methods, tools and techniques to teach and use reflective practice.

This chapter explores and analyses the experiences of five social workers who are using the Fook and Gardner (2007) model of critical reflection, resulting from my interest in exploring critical reflection as a practical and meaningful way of approaching reflective practice that is cognisant with modern workplace demands. I am persuaded by suggestions that critical reflection is a method of advanced reflective practice (Brookfield, 1995; Redmond, 2006; Fook and Gardner, 2007) and is a way to both learn from our experiences and develop our practice in the future. My social work education and practice influenced my decision to recruit social work participants for this research.

Exploring critical reflection

I prefer to remain loyal to the Fook and Gardner (2007) model of critical reflection. Apart from being an acolyte, I have persisted with this model because I have found that it is effective and works for me, and for others. This model provided the structure to help me to identify my values, beliefs and underlying assumptions about my practice as a social worker, and to clarify what was important for me when working with complexity and uncertainty. I learned how to deconstruct my assumptions about uncertainty and change, and I was able to use the critical reflection model to reconstruct my practice in a new, more satisfying way (Hickson, 2011). Critical reflection has been incorporated into my research design and methodology, and I make this point reflexively to acknowledge the influence that critical reflection has on my understanding and interpretations of my research findings.

Study design and method

In this research, I interviewed five social workers, who have been trained in, and use, the Fook and Gardner (2007) model of critical reflection. These social workers have participated in critical reflection training as part of their enrolment in postgraduate study at the Centre for Professional Development, La Trobe University. Apart from their initial training, participants were all involved in both using critical reflection, and teaching critical reflection in formal and informal supervision, including group supervision. There were two male and three female participants who were between forty and sixty years of age. All were experienced social workers with at least ten years of social work experience, and were employed in social work or management roles in public sector or community human service organisations.

This research was a qualitative study, using purposive sampling techniques, and was approved by the La Trobe University Human Research Ethics committee. Social workers were invited to participate in face-to-face or telephone interviews, and interviews were semi-structured with participants asked two broad questions: 'Tell me about your experience of learning about critical reflection' and 'What's been your experience of using critical reflection?'. These questions were designed to explore the participant's individual experience with critical reflection and were followed up with prompt questions as needed. The project was staged over one year, with most participants interviewed twice. Each session was audiotaped (with the participant's consent) and transcribed. Transcripts were then sent to the participant for clarification and approval.

Narrative analysis was used to analyse the data and focus on the way people construct and use stories to interpret their practice. Narrative analysis is a qualitative research method that involves analysis of a person's story or account of their individual experiences (Richmond, 2002; Elliott, 2005). The analysis allows a researcher to understand how participants see things similarly to, and differently from, others, and how the past shapes perceptions of the present and the future. A narrative approach was chosen to access participants' accounts of their experience of learning about and using critical reflection. In addition, Nvivo 8 was used to assist with coding and the identification of themes.

Exploring the experiences of learning and using critical reflection

Whilst exploring the experiences of social workers who use critical reflection, I am aware of the influence of the particular questions that were asked and the ways in which this underpinned the direction of the conversation. In analysing the data for this chapter, I have presented the responses in relation to two main themes: experiences of **learning** critical reflection and experiences of **using** critical reflection. These themes are closely connected and interrelated, and in summary are:

- learning critical reflection
- the importance of journaling
- developing a learned sensitivity to internal triggers
- challenges when learning critical reflection
- importance of understanding the underlying theory
- value of having the process demonstrated by an experienced facilitator
- using critical reflection – deepening understanding of an issue
- integrating critical reflection as a way of being (rather than doing).

Learning critical reflection

Participants in this research study described their experiences of learning about critical reflection as an interesting and exciting, yet sometimes bewildering, adventure. Participants explained how they were drawn to critical reflection because they were looking for both personal and professional challenges, and I was able to deconstruct these experiences of learning about critical reflection with them. What emerged was a focus on the importance of journaling and developing a learned sensitivity to internal triggers.

Importance of journaling

Most participants used written journals while learning critical reflection, and all reported that reading over old journals was helpful and enjoyable. Through exploring this further, I came to understand that the value of journal writing came from the permanent record of reflection that meant that ideas could be 'emptied out of the head' and weren't lost or forgotten. Whilst studying critical reflection as students, participants used a variety of techniques for journal writing, including handwriting on paper, via email or using an electronic journal, and commented on the value of journaling while they were learning how to use critical reflection. Many still had, and treasured, these journals.

Lisa explains:

> The journals were a great way to bring it all together and I was amazed at how quickly the journaling helped me to process things. I stopped writing journals for a while and when I started again, there was so much to let out that I was writing every day. As I was writing, I noticed the decon- struction process started happening very quickly, and the more I wrote the quicker it unpacked – it accelerated the reflection.

Participants discussed the ways they used journal writing to notice themes, explaining that it was helpful to write down their experiences as their memories about an incident changed, and journaling facilitated their remembering at the time of the experience about how they were thinking, feeling and the reasons why they made decisions, how they understood assumptions, and what they perceived other people might be thinking. Through journaling, parti- cipants could read back over their reflections and detect similarities and themes, identify antecedents, and observe how these might have affected outcomes.

This is consistent with Gardner et al.'s (2006), Stuart and Whitmore's (2006) and Bolton's (2010) analyses of the benefits of using writing for critical reflection. Gardner et al. (2006) suggested that deconstructing narratives and focusing on the language used to describe a particular situation can help a person to explore their reaction and assumptions about that time. Stuart and Whitmore (2006) argued that journaling is critical to being able to identify connections between practice intentions and outcomes, and a major tool for deconstructing and understanding reflexivity. Similarly, Bolton's (2010) analysis about the benefits of using a learning journal demonstrated strong empirical value for including journal writing as an aspect of critical reflection.

Developing a learned sensitivity to internal triggers

In my research, journaling was seen as an important way to notice triggers. Triggers were described by one participant as 'the signposts that helped me work out why I took a particular course of action – what I was thinking and feeling and my assumptions about the situation'. Importantly, these journals had also become a tool to keep track of times when participants felt that critical reflection could be used to help resolve a conflict or disparity in expectations. By recording and then deconstructing their reflections, participants reported that they were able to deepen their sensitivity to internal triggers.

It was intriguing to hear participants describe physiological feelings that stimulated them, or reminded them, to use critical reflection to deconstruct or explore their assumptions. The need for describing physiological feelings and physicality has been recognised by Gray (2007), who pointed out that our understanding of our interactions with the world is through our perceptions and senses, including what we see, hear and feel. Gray (2007) argued that critical reflection is perceived too much as a cognitive approach; however, in this research study, participants described physiological and psychological sensations that aroused an internal trigger. They described a gut feeling that triggered an awareness that there was some mismatch of values or assumptions, or something that warranted further exploration. As participants used critical reflection to deconstruct and understand these issues, they reported that they developed sensitivity to their intuition, which was described by Jack as 'tuning in your intuition'. By developing their learned sensitivity to intrusive thoughts, participants were able to learn to recognise times when this could be used to help with problem-solving, rather than it being a feeling to suppress or ignore.

Gayle explained this further:

> I get this feeling in my belly and I think 'Aha – this is when I can use critical reflection to try to work out what's going on here'.

Tina described an uncomfortable feeling that she sometimes experienced when working with her clients that seemed to lead her automatically into using critical reflection:

> I find myself wondering why do I have such a big reaction to this situation? What we are actually doing doesn't sit well with how I understand what we should be doing here? I don't have much of a choice in terms of if I should be doing critical reflection – it follows on automatically.

Jack described that he can feel it in his body – it feels constricting:

> This is a signal to me to stop and have a think about what is happening. Where is this coming from and what are my choices? It's been very empowering to understand this.

This is consistent with Gould and Taylor's (1996) view that reflecting on learning is essential for social work practitioners. Similarly, Maidment and Crisp (2011) suggest that emotion has an impact on reflection and learning, and Kinman and Grant (2011) explain that emotional intelligence can assist social workers to understand and learn from their experiences. Emotional intelligence is attributed to Goleman (1996), who suggested that self-awareness and self-understanding are dependent on emotional intelligence, and argued that people with empathy for others, and the ability to recognise and manage emotions in themselves and others, are better equipped to handle complex relationships and interactions with other people.

Challenges when learning critical reflection

Participants spoke about challenges when learning critical reflection, which include feelings of vulnerability, confusion and unexpected emotions. Jack suggested that the 'muddleness' can be very confronting for people when they are learning critical reflection because:

> we often think that learning is something that should be linear – they teach it, we learn it and away you go. With critical reflection, you are learning a way of thinking, but it's not always clear where you are going and what is at the end. People are sometimes impatient and get lost and frustrated because they want to know where they are going, and I guess that's the very nature of it. People also need to understand that they may experience some personal discomfort and vulnerability thinking about assumptions and values and where they came from.

Brian explained that, in his experience, you need a level of emotional intelligence, an insight into your own emotions, to be able to integrate critical reflection into your practice:

> For people who are action-orientated – the doers – it's a struggle to get them to slow down and think about their practice, and it's also harder for people who aren't open to the possibility of new ideas – they struggle.

Importance of understanding the underlying theory

Participants agreed that the way to overcome these challenges is to take time at the start to understand the theory and the practice of critical reflection. That is, to make sense of the underlying theory about how critical reflection is designed, and the ways in which issues might arise when people begin to examine their assumptions, values, perceptions, thoughts and frustrations. This helps to counter the inevitable need to solve the problem, focusing attention on exploring the assumptions and perceptions that cause the problem to linger.

Value of having the process demonstrated by an experienced facilitator

Participants suggested that it is important to have an experienced facilitator demonstrate the practice of critical reflection. This helps people to understand how the reflection process works and the ways in which issues may be examined. To do this respectfully, it is helpful to allow time for participants to have a think about how, and how much, they want to be involved, and people are able to consider what their options are when they peer into a dark room and feel ready to confront what is inside.

Using critical reflection – deepening understanding of an issue

For three participants, critical reflection provided a technique for deepening their understanding about an issue that was central for them. They spoke about a sense of spiralling around an issue and continually finding their deconstruction of assumptions took them back to familiar territory. This was described as more like a spiral that deepens understanding, rather than a sense of going around in circles and ending up back in the same place. This resonated for me because I continue to have a relationship with uncertainty, and I have wondered if this is because unconsciously I take it back to familiar territory. Through my personal reflection, I have become aware that when there is uncertainty, I may find myself in a place where my assumptions are challenged, and I am conscious that I don't always function at my best when outcomes and expectations change suddenly.

Lisa also identified familiar territory for herself, and spoke about resistance and acceptance as central themes for her. When she uses critical reflection to deconstruct an incident that didn't turn out as well as she had expected, she finds herself exploring her assumptions about resistance and acceptance. Lisa explains that:

> it feels a bit like the eye of a cyclone – where it is calm, but you seem to go around and around but always come back to these central themes. And I wonder what creates this? Is it a life experience that keeps bringing us back to a similar place, and no matter what happens this central theme is going to be there? I have used critical reflection with lots of different groups and different people but I often end up back in familiar territory – the common denominator is me.

Jack spoke about different aspects of his personality – the rebellious child, the responsible social worker and the wise old man – and how critical reflection helped him to understand the different aspects of his thinking and the times when he invited or listened to different voices. Jack was able to recognise times when different aspects of his personality influenced his thinking and decision-making, and he was able to recognise them: 'ah – it's you again'.

Brian disagreed, and suggested that ideas about uncertainty, resistance and acceptance are an entry point rather than a finishing point, commenting: 'my connection to power is a place to rest from which I connect to other things. Maybe it's about different aspects of power – how power is exercised, who has the power, how do people find themselves always resisting power?'.

I have searched through academic literature to find links with other writers about these experiences, and whilst there are links with psychodynamic thinking and spirituality, this is an area of critical reflection that appears to be unexplored.

Integrating critical reflection as a way of being (rather than doing)

Participants in this study talked about critical reflection as a way of being, rather than something that they do. This leaves me wondering: is there a conscious and unconscious aspect to reflection, and how do we integrate critical reflection into professional practice? All participants talked about critical reflection as something that is incorporated into themselves, rather than into work (professional practice) or home (personal), suggesting that it had became 'part of them' and a way of being, rather than something that they needed consciously to remember to do.

Lisa explained:

> the theory and the practice of critical reflection changes the way you see things. I don't have a group of people around me that I can sit down with and deconstruct an incident, but I notice that I use critical reflection all the time. I am on the lookout now for binary language and I can spot it a mile away. I understand power and the way language about power can marginalise people or make them invisible. It becomes integrated into who you are, and I can't 'not think' about things without it. Critical reflection self-talk is a way to keep critical reflection alive – being able to notice what is on the surface and wondering about what might be happening at a deeper level.

Jack agreed and added:

> I see it as a kind of emotional surveillance – a way of thinking about the messages I'm giving people, and how I interpret what I'm getting back from them. I don't work in social work practice any more, but I have found critical reflection almost second nature now – it's not something that I think about doing. It's more about forming the habit of checking assumptions and 'taking for granted' thoughts, and wondering where this is coming from. I have now got an automatic response to checking what I am doing, an automatic way of thinking that puts assumption checking on the radar. It's a default position for me now. I find myself thinking, several times a day, why am I doing this or why am I thinking about this? It's about recognising things around me and the options that I have. I notice the physicality of a constriction in my body and I have options – I can be constricted, or I can make a choice to do something different. It's very liberating. I also notice conversations with other people, when language is filled with binaries, values and assumptions,

and I have a choice about whether to move into that part of the conversation and be more curious, or I might not.

Tina understood this as a reflexive action that happens automatically, and over time helps to build up reflexive thinking:

> It's a bit like building up your muscles. It's not like you have a choice in terms of thinking, should I use critical reflection – it just happens automatically. I'm not always aware of why I have got such a big reaction, but critical reflection gives me a framework to deconstruct what is happening.

This concept has been described by Schön (1983) and Johns (2005) as reflection-in-action. Schön (1983) explains that when people are learning about reflection, they will reflect on their actions after the experience has occurred, and as skills are developed, people will begin to pause during practice to make sense of their situation and work out what to do next. Johns (2005) sees a span of reflection and suggests that, over time, practitioners are able to integrate reflection into a way of being.

Challenges when using critical reflection

Whilst it is understood that learning and using critical reflection are connected and intertwined (Brookfield, 1995; Fook and Gardner, 2007), themes have emerged from this research that may be helpful for those involved in learning, using and teaching critical reflection. Fook and Gardner (2007) describe critical reflection as both a theory and a practice, and neophytes need to appreciate that while it is essential to understand the theory of critical reflection, the process needs to be experienced before the practice can be understood. Alongside this, there needs to be a willingness to be vulnerable and to sit with uncertainty, even though this may be an uncomfortable time, and it cannot be rushed.

Tina explained that, while she can sit comfortably 'not knowing', she sees that a danger of critical reflection is that you can become mired and it can be hard to decide what to do next.

> By analysing your experience and thinking about it from every different perspective, you come up with so many different options that you can feel so lost that you become paralysed and unsure about what to do.

For two participants, the structure of supervision was essential in ensuring that there was a protected time and place for critical reflection to occur. One participant saw their agency management's endorsement of time for a supervision and reflection group as necessary to demonstrate the importance of critical reflection, adding that 'when people get busy the priority for reflection slips, but if the organisation can't make time for reflection to be a priority, then there is a real problem'. Similarly, Lisa explained that she is working in an HR role at the moment and her team and supervisor are not social workers. Lisa has found this to result in a working environment that isn't reflective and where people are focused on the busyness of the job. Lisa explains that she has 'integrated critical reflection into who I am', but at times this leaves her as a lone crusader without a safe environment to be open about what she is thinking and feeling. This is consistent with Baldwin (2004), Reynolds and Vince (2004) and Tosey (2003), who argue that while there are links between individual learning and organisational learning, critical reflection is important for organisations to learn and develop, and this cannot be achieved by individual learning alone.

Areas for closer scrutiny/further research

This leaves me wondering – is there a spectrum of reflection? Is reflection like a pond, with reflection possible at different depths – sometimes warm and shallow; sometimes cool and deep? Where does critical reflection fit in the pond? Does critical reflection occur in the deep part of the pond, where it's not clear what lies beneath? Are there buoys or steps along the way, to guide the reflective practitioner from the shallow end to the deep end, and safely back again? Do we even need this safety net? How do we prepare for ripples and turbulence and manage them when they appear? These are questions for another time, but what is clear is that critical reflection is an effective way for social workers to understand themselves better and to learn from their experiences.

Conclusion

Critical reflection is a valuable tool for social workers to use to reflect on their practice and learn from their experiences. The Fook and Gardner (2007) model of critical reflection can be used in a group supervision context or to assist individual reflection, and is an effective way of deepening understanding about ourselves and our interactions with other people. When learning about critical reflection techniques and methods, journaling is a useful way of noticing and recognising similarities or themes and changes in thinking. By noticing and deconstructing assumptions, workers are able to identify sensations of unease or discomfort and can then recognise, in real time, these sensations to trigger a prompt to reflect on the incident. In my research, participants had integrated critical reflection as a way of being rather than something that you do, and noticing internal triggers is an essential stage in stimulating critical reflection.

References

Baldwin, M. (2004) 'Critical reflection: opportunities and threats to professional learning and service development in social work organizations', in Gould, N. and

Baldwin, M. (eds), *Social Work, Critical Reflection and the Learning Organization*, Aldershot: Ashgate.

Bolton, G. (2010) *Reflective Practice – Writing and Professional Development* (3rd edn), London: Sage.

Brookfield, S. (1995) *Becoming a Critically Reflective Teacher*, San Francisco: Jossey-Bass.

Elliott, J. (2005) *Using Narrative in Social Research. Qualitative and Quantitative Approaches*, London: Sage

Fook, J. and Gardner, F. (2007) *Practising Critical Reflection: A Resource Handbook*, Maidenhead: Open University Press.

Gardner, F., Fook, J. and White, S. (2006) 'Developing effectiveness in conditions of uncertainty', in White, S., Fook, J. and Gardner, F. (eds), *Critical Reflection in Health and Social Care*, Maidenhead: Open University Press.

Goleman, D. (1996) *Emotional Intelligence. Why It Can Matter More Than IQ*, London: Bloomsbury.

Gould, N. and Taylor, I. (eds) (1996) *Reflective Learning for Social Work*, Aldershot: Arena.

Gray, M. (2007) 'The not so critical "critical reflection"', *Australian Social Work*, 60(2): 131–35.

Hickson, H. (2011) 'Critical reflection: reflecting on learning how to be reflective', *Reflective Practice: International and Multidisciplinary Perspectives*, 12(6): 829–39.

Johns, C. (2005) 'Balancing the winds', *Reflective Practice*, 6(1): 67–84.

Kinman, G. and Grant, L. (2011) 'Exploring stress resilience in trainee social workers: the role of emotional and social competencies', *British Journal of Social Work*, 41: 261–75.

Maidment, J. and Crisp, B. (2011) 'The impact of emotions on practicum learning', *Social Work Education*, 30(4): 408–21.

Redmond, B. (2006) *Reflection in Action: Developing Reflective Practice in Health and Social Services* (2nd edn), Aldershot: Ashgate.

Reynolds, M. and Vince, R. (eds) (2004) *Organising Reflection*, Aldershot: Ashgate.

Richmond, H. (2002) 'Learners' lives: a narrative analysis', *The Qualitative Report*, 7(3), www.nova.edu/ssss/QR/QR7-3/richmond.html

Schön, D. (1983) *The Reflective Practitioner – How Professionals Think in Action*, New York: Basic Books.

Stuart, C. and Whitmore, E. (2006) 'Using reflexivity in a research methods course: bridging the gap between research and practice', in White, S., Fook, J. and Gardner, F. (eds), *Critical Reflection in Health and Social Care*, Maidenhead: Open University Press.

Tosey, P. (2003) 'The learning organisation', in Jarvis, P., Holford, J. and Griffin, C. (eds), *The Theory and Practice of Learning* (2nd edn), London: Kogan Page.

6   Using critical reflection to research practice in a mental health setting

Fiona Gardner

Introduction

One of the questions that arises for me in critical reflection training is what is common across disciplines, fields of practice and contexts, and what is different. Much of the writing on critical reflection or reflective practice, including our own, is across disciplines assuming common ground (Rolfe et al., 2011). On the other hand, there is some literature that stresses distinctiveness in a field such as mental health. I have two aims in this chapter: the first is to explore how critical reflection is experienced by practitioners in mental health; the second to identify how critical reflection can be used to research practice, particularly here in relation to supervision.

The chapter focuses on a specific experience of training in critical reflection and supervision in the mental health field in the state of Victoria, Australia. The impetus for the training came from a particular initiative: in 2004, the Department of Human Services instigated the Workforce Development Project, which grouped Victorian mental health services into three clusters. The Western Cluster, which is the one described here, delivers a range of staff development initiatives for staff located in western metropolitan and regional mental health services of Victoria, a large geographical area. In 2008 the Western Cluster Education and Training Unit decided to offer critical reflection and supervision training, initially to social work and occupational therapy staff, and later to other staff from the agencies forming the cluster. I have now run over ten workshops; while all the participants were employed by the same funding body, the staff worked in a variety of contexts, from acute care to community-based support services with young people, families and older people.

I have concentrated here on the initial training with three groups, where the aim was to introduce critical reflection as a possible model for supervision. The way the training was run illustrated how critical reflection could be used to research practice. I have also included findings from five interviews with participants who completed training up to two years ago. What emerges from both the initial training and the interviews is that those in the mental health field have much in common with others in how they perceive and use critical reflection. However, perhaps because of the nature of their work and the related culture, mental health practitioners seem particularly comfortable with the idea of working with unconscious assumptions and values, and are perhaps more used to dealing with emotion and to framing questions sensitively to explore challenging issues.

How the model was used

Initially, the organisers of the training decided that participants needed a general introduction to supervision combined with a focus on training in critical reflection. The expectation was that participants would then either use critical reflection in individual supervision, or develop appropriate group or peer supervision depending on the particular work area. Because of the amount of funding and the numbers of staff interested, it was agreed that there would be a combined first day with about twenty to twenty-five participants. This first day began with a general introduction to supervision, including traditional approaches, current challenges and new ways of thinking about supervision. Essentially, participants were encouraged to think about supervision as a way of exploring 'what do I need to support me in practising well?', rather than as a particular way of connecting with a supervisor.

The second half of the day was essentially the same as the first day of training outlined in Fook and Gardner (2007): the underlying theory and process of critical reflection was presented and discussed, followed by me, as facilitator, presenting an experience of my own which the group then helped me to deconstruct and reconstruct. I deliberately used an experience about supervision. The group then divided in half, with two long half-days of training for each smaller group. Each participant in the group of about ten to twelve participants brought an experience of their own which was then shared and explored in the group – the first half-day for stage one and the second for stage two.

Part of what was distinctive about this training was that I asked all the participants to bring an experience that related to supervision in this organisation, if possible. There were two reasons for this: first, the overall focus of the training was supervision and I thought this would help to generate a shared understanding about supervision issues. Secondly, I wanted to demonstrate how the model could be used to 'research' practice – to build knowledge about how supervision was perceived and operated in the organisation, what was working and what needed to change. In practice, nearly all the participants did bring an experience from their supervision in the agency. My sense is that it helped that I had used an example from my own supervision experience for the demonstration of the process. This example described a situation where I had misinterpreted a worker's enjoyment of what she called 'drama in her life' as her being stressed. The exploration of this made it clear that I was prepared to engage with my 'failure' as a supervisor and to challenge my own assumptions about my desire to be the perfect supervisor and my acceptance of difference.

In the second and third sessions, because of the agenda about researching practice, once each individual had reached clarity for themselves, we then as a group noted what the experience suggested about supervision in the organisation and its culture – in the first stage, both what was working well and existing dilemmas and issues; in the second, what to change and how to change it. The value of this became clearer over the course of the training. Each experience contributed more 'knowledge' that could be used to build a more complex picture of how supervision practises. By the end of the third session, participants were able to identify the underlying values and assumptions related to supervision in the organisation, as well as for themselves individually, and as a group. They had also articulated aspects of supervision that were working well and other aspects that needed to change, and generated some ideas about how those changes could come about.

Assumptions related to professional practice, and about practice within organisations, in this setting

I am focusing here on the responses from the groups that relate to supervision. The implications of these will be explored further later in this chapter. Participants identified a wide range of assumptions that were perceived as positive or helpful, as well as many others that were unhelpful. The process was that we initially identified any assumptions that people had about supervision, then over the process of the workshops we modified or added to these so that they could become positive principles from which to operate. Those identified here are assumptions that have been considered to be useful principles to work from.

- Supervision can be rewarding/positive – you learn from someone you supervise.
- Supervisors will vary, have different levels of skill, training and insight.
- Supervision can be a way of seeing people grow their skills.
- Supervision is energising when it makes internal values external and enables experiences to be used constructively.
- Supervisors can be agents of change/be powerful, and need to be strategic agents of change.
- Supervisors need to be themselves – to acknowledge what they can and can't do.
- Supervision can have an impact on stress levels – positive and negative.
- It is important to start supervision well, with expectations and ground rules, to have a process to fix things, and to acknowledge what can and can't be fixed and where to go.
- Supervision match is not always perfect, but can be magic – there is a need to work on who can provide what in supervision.
- Supervisors, as well as supervisees, have needs and it is reasonable for them to be expressed.

- Supervision needs to change to fit changing supervision needs. We all have the right to ask for the supervision we want/need.
- Differences in power need to be acknowledged. Supervisors need to recognise their own issues/potential of power to be used negatively.
- Effective supervision is a shared responsibility – there is a need for a collaborative approach, co-creation or co-construction, while acknowledging power differences and accountability.
- Good supervisors give people an opportunity to change – choice, not telling.
- Supervisors are human and not perfect (grey is okay); not knowing can be positive. Supervisors won't always be right – more important is commitment to working on mistakes/issues, reaching closure where possible.
- Expressing emotion and vulnerability appropriately can be a way to move forward – to own one's feelings of being stuck or frustrated.
- Silence can be helpful in supervision.
- There are many ways for supervision to be provided – there is a need to look for creative possibilities such as using other workers for specific issues, critical reflection forums, external supervision, peer groups.
- Supervisors can be the role model for self-care, recognising that self-care is both personal and professional.
- Supervisors need to be clear that it is okay to say that some behaviour/ attitudes are *not* okay.

These assumptions or principles were new for many participants, and indicated new possibilities for attitudes and behaviour. For some it was liberating to embrace the idea that they did not have to be perfect, that they too were learning from the experience. Many found it transforming to see how to name what was happening in a way that could open up possibilities for discussion rather than suggesting blame: accepting differences in personality, assumptions or style rather than thinking there had to be one 'right' way.

A number of the assumptions related to what was identified as a dilemma or tension in the organisation: the influence of the prevailing more managerial culture which was sometimes experienced as epitomising different values from a clinical approach. Some staff in the organisation had two managers. The first was generally a line or accountability manager, who was not necessarily from the same discipline and who was responsible for such issues as quality of work and compliance with organisational standards. Sometimes participants felt there was a conflict between espoused theory and theory in practice for their line managers: for example, in saying that difference should be affirmed, but on the other hand supporting organisational rules that made this very difficult. The second type of supervisor – often called a clinical supervisor – generally came from the same discipline and was responsible for what is called in the literature enabling or restorative supervision (Kadushin, 1985; Proctor, 2008). These different approaches were sometimes experienced as being complementary, but at other times as conflicting, as expressed in the following assumptions:

- there's more to mental health supervision than tasks – ice plus berg
- mental health clinicians are more comfortable with uncertainty, with relatedness and process than their managers who are part of the dominant culture
- the clinical side is less powerful, but more comfortable with uncertainty, with relatedness, process, slower, more personal risk.

In relation to this potential tension with line managers, one group identified the following assumptions:

- may not be 'psychodynamically minded'
- some well defended, not prepared to get other view
- there are different strategies and different resistances – need to check language and try other things, explore what turns person into turtle.

Some also felt that assumptions embedded in the broader structural context had an influence on their practice in mental health, such as mixed messages about the value of self-care versus the need to achieve outcomes; focus on career rather than skill development. This included a focus on finance, management and outcomes, rule compliance – 'forget the berg, the ice is the important bit'. Some considered this to be a tension for at least some managers as well, influenced by government funding reflecting society not seeing mental health or illness as important. The impact of power relationships was seen as central: one group particularly questioned the influence of gender and culture on styles of expression.

My observations

It was quickly evident that critical reflection was a way of understanding, processing and changing practice that was congruent with working in mental health, and this is confirmed in the feedback explored later in this chapter. Much of the feedback was consistent with that of other fields of practice, so here I concentrate on the aspects of this experience that were distinctive.

I was interested that mental health practitioners seemed particularly comfortable with the idea of working with the unconscious, an essential part of critical reflection that some participants struggle with. Many participants were accustomed to identifying underlying feelings and thoughts and making these conscious – their own as well as their clients' – and often identified experience in psychodynamic thinking as part of this. They were particularly tuned in to exploring parallels in processes: how the interactions between clients and workers mirrored those between workers and supervisors, supervisors and managers. This was also implicit in the language used: for example, as well as naming psychodynamic ideas as useful, they questioned whether an individual (manager, supervisee or client) was defended or defensive, resistant or mindful. The critical reflection process of also unearthing assumptions from all parties – their own as well as those of clients, other colleagues, managers and the organisation – reinforced and, for some, sharpened their ability to do this, but also took it to another level. Participants felt critical reflection extended their thinking about underlying assumptions and values to seeing the influence of the broader social context.

Mental health practitioners were also particularly conscious of the importance of engaging with emotions; some connected this again to their familiarity with psychodynamic ways of working. For example, they readily acknowledged the vulnerability that comes from shared emotion for both the asker and the asked. They noted the value of tears, a symbol of the emotion, and the need to explore what this meant. The value of acknowledging and validating feelings first, then exploring processes that lead to change, was identified as important in their work with clients, and they recognised the centrality of this in the critical reflection process. They identified what Huffington et al. (2004: 3), using a psychoanalytic approach, call 'working below the surface' of organisational life, identifying the emotions that are influencing organisational interactions and processes.

This group of mental health practitioners were also fluent in noticing and working with language – how ideas and feelings were expressed – and pursuing these to deconstruct and reconstruct. They were adept at developing and then actively using illuminating metaphors to extend understanding. For example, one person talked about themselves as being 'like a dog with a bone'. Others took this up and explored the need to be 'aware of your own bones', a helpful link to the dangers of not recognising your own assumptions and values and the danger of wanting to project these onto others. Similarly, the iceberg metaphor, which started as a way of naming the desire to look more deeply at what is happening under the surface, what is unconscious, became a way of exploring differences in supervision and management.

Some of those in the groups also commented specifically about the value of social work training and experience, suggesting that this had helped them firstly in being reflective, but also in remembering the importance of social context. There was a view that this also enabled them to engage more easily with critical reflection. I was interested in this comment, partly because some similar comments had been made in other organisations. This is not to say that all social workers would agree, or that those in other professions are less able to critically reflect, but it might suggest the value of including this in professional training.

Finally, using the critical reflection process to 'research practice' was very effective and could be used in a variety of ways in organisations. Participants valued the opportunity to reflect more formally on their own reactions to each person's experience and to explore similarities and differences about (in this example) supervision. Given that time was tight, this discussion had to remain focused. In spite of this, collectively, the discussion led to a rich exchange of views and the generation of knowledge that could be used in practice.

Evaluations of critical reflection: impact on practice

I have combined here the results from a follow-up session with the three groups described above, which happened six months to a year after initial training, with the findings from five interviews with those who completed training in later sessions.

Both included asking what difference critical reflection had made to practice and what had helped the process to work. Most participants were using critical reflection in individual supervision; some had initiated peer supervision groups, including groups of those who had completed training together. What people identified included the following.

Becoming critically reflective

What people meant by this was being conscious of the value of critical reflection, and looking for both formal and informal opportunities to use it. This might mean a supervisee being in a reflective mood either in supervision or during a brief conversation. What was significant here was maintaining consciousness of using critical reflection, with clients or colleagues seeing it as a fundamental part of practice. As one participant said: 'This is hard in some ways to identify as it is so integral to everything I do.' For some, this included thinking about the organisation and policy context as well as client work.

Sitting with the unknown and uncertain

This was often viewed as being prepared to talk about what is unfamiliar territory, while acknowledging each other's existing knowledge and experience. The attitude was of being involved in learning at the same time, seeing this as a joint endeavour and sharing power. Some participants talked about a shift in attitude from tending to steer conversations in a particular way, a more problem-solving approach, to allowing people to 'talk about what they want even if it seems off track', or having an attitude of 'curiosity' and openness to conversations and interviews. This often opened up other ways in which issues and relationships could be seen. What helped was partly a shift in attitude, and partly simply asking more open and more critically reflective questions. Some commented that the critical reflection training had enabled them to see how to ask questions in a more open way.

Acknowledging difference

This was a theme that ran through all the other areas – identifying and valuing difference. Participants could see that accepting their differences was congruent with effective work, such as some people talking to gain clarity, or others needing quiet. Taking this on board was helpful in allowing self and others to be different. For some, seeing different perspectives related to the following.

Remembering the broader context

For some this was primarily organisational, for others it included both the organisation and the broader social culture. One participant named this as 'trying to think bigger'; others felt prompted to remember the influence on themselves and their clients of the social culture and prevailing attitudes about mental illness. Having such awareness included being active about seeking change in the broader context: either organisationally, in changes in attitudes, actions or policies; or in the wider culture, such as in challenging being considered strange to enjoy working with people with mental illness.

More collaborative relationships

Valuing diversity also linked to developing more collegiate or collaborative relationships. Being more aware of others' perspectives and how they might differ from one's own generated deeper, shared understanding and, contrary to what might be expected, greater capacity to work together. The expectation was that everyone involved needed to be aware of their own reactions and reflections and able to feed these back into the session or a working relationship when appropriate. This was seen as generating a more shared sense of work.

Creating a safe space for reflection

The importance of a safe space was raised by many participants. Ruch (2007) affirms the need for such safety, given the need to sit with uncertainty, as mentioned above, and the anxiety that results from this. She suggests the value of Bion's concept of containment to generate thinking for individuals, teams and the organisation about how to allow safe expression and exploration of emotion.

The development of an example of a safe space in training contributed to awareness of how this could and should happen for supervision. Part of this was accepting that one person's perception of safety might not be the same as another's and being prepared to negotiate. Principles such as validation of the person (for both supervisor and/or supervisee), transparency and honesty, and a sense of reciprocity were all identified as important in creating a safe space for reflection.

Impact on organisational context

Participants noted that their own internal changes would also have an impact on the organisation. More formally, there were two main new assumptions that related to change. First, 'supervision is a negotiated package'. This shifted the sense of power in relation to supervision from 'this is decided by other people' to 'this is something that I too can influence'. This included views that supervision works better if prepared and purposeful, if the person is valued and there is time for reflection before and in the sessions, that supervision tunes into the whole person and is about quality and depth of reflection rather than a task focus.

A second assumption that complemented this was that culture is important, and therefore that supervisor and supervisee need to work to change the organisation. Participants felt it was important to move beyond binaries of analysis versus action, or process versus outcome, and to see how these could combine. They were able to come up with some specific suggestions about how to do this. For example, a frequent suggestion about managing tensions between managerial and more clinical approaches was simply to name the issue and explore it as a team or with a particular manager.

There was also a range of suggestions about what to do about identified problems with supervision more generally. For example, strategies were identified about planning for interim supervision, to have better orientation to supervision, and to seek acceptance that people could choose their own supervisors to a greater degree. The initial groups also decided to establish their own peer supervision groups.

More specifically in relation to critical reflection, participants felt that it would be important to use critical reflection and practise it in their own individual supervision first. For those whose supervisors had not done the training, this included needing to educate up and to affirm that this way of going about supervision would be important across teams. They also thought it was important to practise being a facilitator for critical reflection both in their individual supervision with supervisees or supervisors, and in generating peer supervision using this model and so becoming a reflective team.

Where to from here?

The experience of the participants confirms the value of using critical reflection in mental health settings. Participants identified the appeal of a critical reflection framework that enabled them to explore their practice more deeply, reinforcing the capacity to work with the 'berg' – the underlying and unconscious assumptions, values and feelings that influence practice with clients and in supervision. Critical reflection was also helpful in reminding participants of the 'bigger picture' structural issues influencing them.

The experience here also highlights how critical reflection can be used to research practice in the sense of identifying the knowledge that is inherent in practice experience and wisdom. Participants in the training groups were able to tease out in depth those aspects that worked (so needed to be nurtured) as well as internal tensions within the organisation that could work against effective supervision. Recognising their collective knowledge enabled participants to develop constructive and realistic plans about how to increase the value of supervision for individuals, teams and the organisation. Part of what was significant was developing greater understanding of the organisational culture combined with a sense of agency about changing it individually and collectively.

Working with this group of mental health practitioners also reinforced the sense that different fields of practice and/or disciplines have differences in their culture which may influence their experience of critical reflection. The literature has tended to focus on different aspects of this: some writers in the mental health field would argue for reflective practice with a psychoanalytical approach, given the complex dynamics of work with individuals and families (Webber and Nathan, 2010). On the other hand, Crowe and O'Malley (2006), also focusing on mental health, affirm the importance of awareness of the social context that critical thinking encourages. Others would stress the importance of a critically reflective approach in generating cultural competence in mental health, with critical reflexivity being seen as an essential part of culturally safe practice (Walker and Sonn, 2010). The increased interest in mindfulness as a therapeutic approach (Hick, 2008: 7) is another aspect of the mental health field that may influence, and be influenced by, a critically reflective approach: a way of encouraging a more contemplative stand and resisting the 'results-oriented society'. What does seem to be agreed in the literature is that mental health practice is faced with increasing complexity which requires 'advanced' practitioners able to think and reflect on their practice at deeper levels (Crowe and O'Malley, 2006; Nathan, 2010).

For the practitioners identified in this chapter, it seemed that critical reflection provided both the theory and the process to face such complexity and reflect more deeply. Familiarity with ideas about the unconscious from psychodynamic theory helped predispose them to actively unearth their own emotions, assumptions and values as part of the critical reflection process. Knowledge of other psychodynamic concepts of projection, defences and resistance also contributed to seeing how an individual might, or might not, engage with the process. This suggests the value in training of being conscious of what is particular about the culture and practice theory of an organisation or discipline in order to incorporate and build on what is known.

Clearly, critical reflection is predicated on an understanding that practitioners are operating from what is unconscious or implicit, and the advantages of making this conscious or explicit, articulating what Mezirow, from an adult learning perspective, calls 'meaning perspectives' or 'frames of reference' (Mezirow, 2000: 16). However, writing about critical reflection has tended to see psychodynamic thinking as too individually focused, and a similar comment can be made about reflective practice. Brookfield (2009: 293) points out that 'reflection is not by definition critical' unless it is explicitly questioning the dynamics of power and ingrained social assumptions. Ruch (2009) affirms the value of psychodynamic thinking more generally in 'relationship-based practice' while also acknowledging the need for this to be complemented by critical thinking. She suggests the need to move beyond the binary thinking that stresses the differences to seeing what is common, such as 'commitment to complexity within a wider socio-political context', and suggests a relationship-based model of reflection that enables participants to address issues of power. Perhaps what needs to be included more here is the complexities of power as explored in critical social theory: how power relationships at a structural level are internalised by individuals, creating the need for change at multiple levels. As with any other theory, then there are questions to explore about the potential for psychodynamic thinking to complement a critically reflective approach.

What is clear from this chapter is the value of a critically reflective approach in a mental health setting, both as a general sense of reflecting critically on practice, and also as a way to 'research practice', focusing on a particular area to articulate practice knowledge. The key here is remembering the *critical* aspect of critical reflection: continuing to make connections between the conscious and the unconscious, the individual and the wider social context, and actively and consciously seeking change.

References

Brookfield, S. (2005) *The Power of Critical Theory: Liberating Adult Learning and Teaching*, San Francisco: Jossey-Bass.
——(2009) 'The concept of critical reflection: promises and contradictions', *European Journal of Social Work*, 12(3): 293–304.
Crowe, M.T. and O'Malley, J. (2006) 'Teaching critical reflection skills for advanced mental health nursing practice: a deconstructive–reconstructive approach', *Journal of Advanced Nursing*, 56(1): 79–87.
Fook, J. and Gardner, F. (2007) *Practising Critical Reflection: A Resource Handbook*, Maidenhead: Open University Press.
Hick, S.F. (2008) 'Cultivating therapeutic relationships: the role of mindfulness', in Hick, S.F. and Bien, T. (eds), *Mindfulness and the Therapeutic Relationship*, New York/London: Guilford Press, 1–17.
Huffington, C., Armstrong, D., Halton, W., Hoyle, L. and Pooley, J. (2004) *Working Below the Surface: The Emotional Life of Contemporary Organizations*, London: Karnac.
Kadushin, A. (1985) *Supervision in Social Work*, New York: Columbia University Press.
Mezirow, J. (ed.) (2000) *Learning as Transformation*, San Francisco, CA: Jossey-Bass.
Nathan, J. (2010) 'The making of the advanced practitioner in social work', in Webber, M. and Nathan, J. (eds), *Reflective Practice in Mental Health: Advanced Psychosocial Practice*, London: Jessica Kingsley, 29–43.
Proctor, B. (2008) *Group Supervision: A Guide to Creative Practice*, London: Sage.
Rolfe, G.M., Jasper, M. and Freshwater, D. (2011) *Critical Reflection in Practice: Generating Knowledge for Care*, Houndmills: Palgrave Macmillan.
Ruch, G. (2007) 'Reflective practice in child-care social work: the role of containment', *British Journal of Social Work*, 37(4): 659–80.
——(2009) 'Identifying "the critical" in a relationship-based model of reflection', *European Journal of Social Work*, 12(3): 349–62.

Walker, R. and Sonn, C. (2010) 'Working as a culturally competent mental health practitioner', in Purdie, N., Dudgeon, P. and Walker, R. (eds), *Working Together: Aboriginal and Torres Strait Islander Health and Wellbeing Principles and Practice*, Canberra: Australian Government for Health and Ageing, 157–80.

Webber, M. and Nathan, J. (2010) *Reflective Practice in Mental Health: Advanced Psychosocial Practice*, London: Jessica Kingsley.

Section 2

Critical reflection in supervision and management

7   Critical reflection in statutory work

Yolande Ferguson

This chapter explores the use of the Fook/Gardner model for critical reflection as used to support groups of newly qualified social workers (NQSWs) as well as residential workers from a children's home.

The model of critical reflection used

I have been implementing critical reflection to be used in groups with NQSWs working in statutory children and family teams in a West London Local Authority (UK) as well as with a staff group of residential support workers (RSWs) with supervisory responsibilities from a children's home within the Local Authority.

The Local Authority is currently running a pilot NQSW programme to support NQSWs working in children and families social work teams across the borough. One of the provisions of this programme has been to provide NQSWs with facilitated critical reflection sessions on a monthly basis. I have previously run one group for all NQSWs and, together with two colleagues, am currently running three smaller groups for the present cohort of NQSWs.

The staff group of RSWs with supervisory responsibilities had previously attended critical reflection training aimed at supporting them to develop a more critically reflective approach to managing supervision of staff.

How this differs from the Fook/Gardner 2007 model

All the critical reflection group sessions with NQSWs have been based specifically on the Fook/Gardner 2007 model for group critical reflection as outlined in Fook and Gardner (2007). Initially the sessions were divided so that in each monthly session one NQSW would complete a stage 1 reflection and another would do their stage 2 reflection (having completed their stage 1 in the month before). This was motivated by Fook and Gardner (2007) stating that 'We think it important to separate the two stages of critical reflection on assumptions and critical reflection on changed assumptions and practices.' It was felt that the month between critical reflection sessions would offer significant space during which the NQSWs could consider their stage 1 reflection before then participating in the stage 2 reflection.

Practical issues arose that presented obstacles to following the initial format for the groups described. An ongoing obstacle to consistent implementation of the format was that many NQSWs are based in busy frontline social work teams, where matters relating to child protection and court proceedings often had to be prioritised, and group members therefore could not attend critical reflection sessions. This meant that some NQSWs did not complete their stage 2 reflection until much later, or NQSWs who were present for a stage 1 were not present for a group member's stage 2 and *vice versa*. This created a detached group dynamic, where group members were not realistically following the critical reflection group format in a meaningful way that could consistently make sense of discussions and generate substantial facilitative questions or a sense of shared learning.

Fook and Gardner (2007) note that the culture of the group is important in sustaining the appropriate process, and in this case the inconsistent attendance of NQSWs affected the opportunity to develop more meaningful group dynamics, which has in turn hindered the chance of fostering an ongoing learning process for the group as a whole. In order to overcome this issue, the critical reflection group format for NQSWs was altered so that the NQSW presenting their critical incident would complete their stage 1 and their stage 2 in the same session, with the two stages separated by a break in the middle. The revised format has ensured that NQSWs presenting a critical incident are facilitated through their stage 1 and stage 2 reflection within the one group session. This has provided the opportunity for the NQSW to have a more complete critical reflection experience; however, the sporadic nature of attendance by group members continued. Although the changed format allowed for a more complete reflection, it did not necessarily equate to a more cohesive group dynamic that would be expected to form as a result of regular ongoing attendance by all group members. I believe that the group culture begins to grow and develop from the moment the group members first meet, and so when social workers are unable to attend a group session regularly, the group in a sense struggles to take off as it consists of different members from one month to the next.

A further issue that has arisen due to the sporadic attendance of group members has been that the initial introduction of the critical reflection group process was disjointed. Group members received the introduction, including theoretical underpinnings and process, in a fragmented fashion bound by time constraints. This was a significant issue throughout the first NQSW group that was run. A core group of three social workers received the introduction to the critical reflection group process and continued attending regularly, whilst other group members attended sporadically throughout the group's continuation. This ongoing pattern resulted in a group dynamic where some group members appeared fully engaged and participative, whilst others continued to appear less confident with the process. Current groups have had a more thorough introduction to the group process with all or the majority of participants present, which appears to have contributed positively to group cohesion and a shared experience of learning.

The critical reflection sessions with RSWs have from the start been based on the amended group format discussed previously, where stage 1 and stage 2 reflections are completed within the same session. Sessions with RSWs have not run as frequently as those with NQSWs, and so the decision to keep the stages within the same session was taken to ensure that RSWs had the opportunity to complete the full reflection. Practically, this was also structured with the RSW undergoing a stage 1 reflection followed by a break before starting their stage 2 reflection, which allows for some separation of stages.

Assumptions that emerged regarding professional practice and about practice within organisations

Throughout my experience of facilitating critical reflection groups, the process has uncovered several important assumptions by group participants and I, too, have discovered some of my own assumptions about professional social work practice and about practice within organisations.

When I started facilitating critical reflection groups, I made the assumption that NQSWs would attend the sessions and find them helpful, as they would appreciate the need to reflect and the need to take responsibility for reflecting on one's own practice. I have, however, since discovered that however committed an NQSW may intend to be to a group critical reflection process, they are often under significant pressures relating to everyday practice that can create obstacles to attending critical reflection group sessions. Donnellan and Jack (2010: 94) acknowledge the reality that social work is a busy and pressurised job, and so many social workers feel that the usual working day often does not provide enough time for meeting all the necessary demands placed on them. When considering why NQSWs have struggled with regular attendance, I appreciate the need to take into account the immense pressure under which social workers operate on a daily basis due to the expectations of needing to prioritise statutory duty and duties to protect children.

Donnellan and Jack (2010: 108) also talk about the shock experienced by new entrants to the social work profession when the tensions between ideal and real practice begin to manifest themselves almost immediately. This is perhaps a view that could explain some of the overwhelming pressure that NQSWs may be experiencing when they are struggling to prioritise ideal practice experience, such as regular attendance at critical reflection groups, versus the need to prioritise statutory duties and tasks. This has particularly been evident in relation to NQSWs from frontline teams where the pressure of child protection is at times exceedingly time-consuming and stressful for even the most experienced social workers. Donnellan and Jack (2010: 39) acknowledge the importance of saying 'no' in a busy, pressurised workplace, and the fact that for NQSWs it can be particularly difficult to say 'no' when they are trying to prove their enthusiasm and commitment to the job and so they are tempted to accept every task offered. It may be that the challenge of saying 'no' has been a relevant issue that has meant several NQSWs have found themselves busy beyond the point of being able to prioritise attending the critical reflection groups.

In terms of frequency of attendance, I have noticed some differences between attendance of NQSWs who have previously been working in unqualified roles, such as family support workers and personal advisors within the field of social care, and those NQSWs who have no prior experience of working within social care on a full-time basis. Generally, the NQSWs with prior experience of working in the field of social care have attended critical reflection sessions on a more regular basis. I initially assumed that this was perhaps reflective of these NQSWs being more enthusiastic or appreciative of the need for critical reflection; however, I have realised that their more regular attendance could perhaps be a reflection of these NQSWs having more experience of saying 'no' and perhaps feeling less pressure to prove themselves now, as qualified workers, and therefore being more confident to prioritise attending the group session.

Due to the above attendance trends, I had wondered whether it was perhaps more realistic to deliver the critical reflection group sessions to a target group who were more likely to attend. This consideration was also brought about by the fact that I have had numerous comments from managers at various levels, as well as experienced social workers, questioning why NQSWs have access to critical reflection groups but not them. I wondered whether their enthusiasm was perhaps an indication of a group of workers who might more readily receive and attend the critical reflection group process.

In order to support attendance and make critical reflection sessions more readily available to all NQSWs, including those struggling to prioritise attendance, the decision was made to develop three area-based groups. This has ensured that sessions are more easily accessible and NQSWs are not needing to take extra time out to travel to and from critical reflection sessions.

One of the issues that has arisen for NQSWs without prior experience of working within social work settings has been the challenge of entering a workplace where they feel all those around them appear to know what they are doing and function with a sense of confidence that they do not them-selves intrinsically feel – they can at times feel weighed down by their own expectations of needing to perform well and produce a standard of work that equates to the calibre of the more experienced members of their team. It may be that this is a reflection of Donnellan and Jack's (2010: 27–30, 183) description of NQSWs undergoing the 'novice' learner phase of developing from having technical knowledge of context-free rules as a student, to gradually modifying and adapting these rules in light of experience in different situa-tions in the workplace to become 'situational' rules founded on practical knowledge and know-how. As the NQSWs enter practice, they have not yet developed advanced situational understanding or context for their social work knowledge, and therefore can feel overwhelmed by the more experienced workers around them appearing a lot more confident, with more experience and skills for functioning independently and in a manner that appears more efficient, than how NQSWs feel about their own practice.

A theme that has perhaps been the most common to arise during critical reflection sessions with NQSWs has been about assumptions that social work would offer the opportunity to help and support people in a positive way that would be pleasant and rewarding to carry out. NQSWs have reflected experiences of feeling disillusioned with bureaucracy and the stressful nature of statutory and frontline social work responsibilities. In relation to this issue, NQSWs have often noted a struggle with the realisation that the process of helping is not always an enjoyable or rewarding one, and can at times be emotionally painful for both them and their service users. Feelings of disillusionment have at times been connected to NQSWs facing the realities of how financial restrictions and bureaucratic procedures can present frustrating obstacles in the course of fulfilling social work duties in the ultimate manner. NQSWs resultantly feel that they cannot do the job as they had ideally thought they would, and feel disheartened by their new perception of statutory social work, as well as about the service that service users are receiving. Donnellan and Jack (2010: 109) talk about these issues, combined with low social recognition and poor regard for the profession, as factors frequently identified by social workers as sources of stress.

In addition to low social recognition, Donnellan and Jack (2010: 109) also highlight how media portrayals and political criticisms of social work incompetence lead to feelings of being undervalued and misunderstood, compared with other professionals working with children and young people. Related assumptions about how social workers feel British society views them have been a common theme among NQSWs who have previously worked in other unqualified roles within the field of social work. These NQSWs have previously held support roles, such as family support workers and personal advisors, and found that they had generally been welcomed as the 'supporting person'; however, as social workers with statutory duties to intervene where children and families are at risk, the NQSWs are discovering that they are no longer viewed in the same way as a 'helper', but rather as 'trouble' or an unwelcome presence. This realisation has been a theme within critical incidents discussed during critical reflection sessions, and has uncovered feelings of insecurity and dissatisfaction in relation to assumptions about how NQSWs feel they are now being viewed as a social worker as opposed to their previous helping or supporting roles which service users more gladly accepted.

Critical reflection sessions with RSWs enabled them to uncover personal assumptions that they have made about each other. Participants felt that by supporting colleagues to reflect on their critical incidents, they were able to better understand their colleagues' personalities, as well as the related motivations for the perceived behaviours of colleagues. Lawson (2002) talks about the interdependency of staff teams working in group care as opposed to field work: in group care the whole team will work with all the service users on both an individual and a group basis. Lawson (2002) also acknowledges that the functioning of the staff team is therefore of particular importance, as difficulties within the team will be played out in various ways through the work of the unit. This has been echoed in the reflections of RSWs who have recognised how assumptions and resultant misunderstandings among staff can at times derail focus and create tensions that hinder the course of delivering best possible services. RSWs have significantly valued the opportunity to understand RSW colleagues better, and this has led to increased tolerance and motivation to want to work together positively to achieve shared goals for the service.

This has led me to believe that the group format of critical reflection may be one that, if carried out appropriately, could offer the opportunity for team-building and improved communication and dynamics within a team. I have supported the implementation session of group critical reflection in a different London local authority, where critical reflection group sessions will be run within teams. One of the aims for this work, aside from improving practice, is to develop team cohesion and teamwork.

Observations about the use of critical reflection

Lawson (2002) explains that work in residential settings involves prolonged contact with service users who will have experienced loss and may be frightened, angry or distressed, so the work involves attention to the residents' emotional and physical needs. Lawson acknowledges that if staff are to be equipped to work effectively with others' distress, they need to have an understanding of the support mechanisms available to them, good self-knowledge, and a supportive structure with high-quality supervision. Initially, the RSW group spoke about wanting to develop their supervision skills, because at times during supervision they have found it challenging to provide their supervisees with an appropriate balance of being emotionally supportive whilst also addressing performance issues. Participants within the RSW group have acknowledged the value of, through the critical reflection group process, learning to ask exploratory questions in a non-judgemental way. They have come to realise that learning to ask questions without judgement or validation is important in order to be able to use a style of communication that builds a foundation on which to talk about difficult and often painful issues. RSWs have also learnt that a non-judgemental as well as non-affirming approach to exploring issues with supervisees will enhance the supervisee's ability to explore and reflect on critical incidents or issues in a manner through which they can optimally learn and develop a better understanding of their behaviour, as well as identify ways to improve their practice in the future. A non-judgemental approach ensures the supervisee does not instinctively respond in a defensive manner that would inhibit more meaningful, open reflection; a non-affirming approach ensures the supervisee's reflection is not abandoned prematurely if validation results in feeling that, as their supervisor agrees with them, they are correct in their thinking and thus further reflection seems unnecessary.

RSWs acknowledged that they had realised the importance of listening well, as it was only through attentive listening that they felt confident they were asking relevant questions to facilitate individuals' reflection. By being non-judgemental and developing good listening skills, RSWs have learned an approach that can help ensure their supervisees feel understood and supported when personal issues or difficulties arise, as for example when working within an emotional environment that stirs up their own issues.

Similarly to RSWs, NQSWs have also acknowledged the benefit of the critical reflection group process providing an opportunity to become more confident in using non-judgemental and open questions, which has in practice provided improved communication skills with which to be able to explore difficult issues with service users. Personally, I have also found this useful within my own practice with service users as well as while supervising staff. The ability to develop a language for asking difficult questions so as not to offend or cause distress for the recipient has provided a practical tool for supporting better practice with service users, colleagues and other professionals.

One staff member from the children's home advised that they felt reflection about critical incidents at work had enabled them to understand better how childhood experiences have influenced their current functioning within their professional life, which they feel is valuable and integral to their personal and professional development.

Some NQSWs have made comments that the process of group critical reflection has enabled them to accept or understand that it is okay not to 'have all the answers' or to know everything from the start. The opportunity to share experiences with other NQSWs within a group format has supported NQSWs to feel less isolated and to realise that, as an NQSW, it is natural and acceptable to be at a heightened phase of learning and you are not expected to know everything. Jackson (2007) acknowledges the importance of understanding ourselves so that we can identify the difference between our own responses from those of our service users. Often, service users can make demands or have expectations that are unrealistic or not achievable, and in order to try to meet their expectations, as social workers we can lose ourselves or feel lost in a situation that appears to have no resolution. NQSWs have echoed that critical reflection has enabled them to see themselves and the social work task as two separate parts. They have found it helpful to reflect in a manner that has made greater sense of the differentiation between assumed expectations, either self-assumed or assumed by service users, and the reality of what can reasonably be expected of them based on resources available and realities of social work statutory responsibilities.

Many social work principles support service user empowerment. I find it interesting that, as social workers, we often associate the concept of empowerment with ways in which we approach and work with service users; however, perhaps we do not pay as much attention to the need for social workers to be empowered in order to be able to do our job effectively. Howe (2009) states that working with others who share the same need or experience, or suffer the same oppression, is an effective way of helping people become aware of their situation. If we support social work service users to develop support networks and engage in services that understand their situation, why would we as social workers not do the same for ourselves? We can access support through group critical reflection facilitated by colleagues who understand our situations and experiences.

Munro (2011) acknowledges that being exposed to powerful and often negative emotions experienced in child protection can come at a personal cost to workers. She notes that if the work environment does not help to support workers and debrief them from traumatic experiences, then it increases the probability of staff burnout. It is my experience that the Fook/ Gardner model for critical reflection offers a facilitated group process that can help social workers make sense of their negative emotions and move past the feelings that can stifle them. I believe this can be empowering for social workers. This is also echoed by Howe (2009): 'Things that make sense can be controlled. To be in control of a difficult experience is empowering.'

The group model also ensures a non-judgemental environment, which is in itself empowering for social workers who often experience the stress of working within a culture of blame. Munro (2011) has acknowledged in her review of child protection that social workers experience anxiety about being blamed. I feel that the non-judgemental climate offered during group critical reflection supports social workers to explore and reflect on their critical experiences more freely as the context of blame has been removed. This can be very empowering and uplifting, and although the focus is not on validating or affirming the specific practice of the worker, they can often come away from the experience feeling positive about focusing on their own self-identified plan for improved practice. They can own the plan and feel empowered by recognising that they have independently identified a way to improve their practice, which can also build self-confidence.

Evaluations and results

The primary form of evaluating critical reflection to date has been through open dialogue and written feedback. Not all NQSWs have responded to the request for feedback; however, all RSWs responded. Generally, the staff who have attended critical reflection sessions regularly are the ones who have provided more feedback.

Impact on practice/organisational context

Following the process of completing stage 1 and stage 2 reflections, NQSWs generally agreed that they felt less stuck within the difficulties of the critical issues on which they were reflecting. One NQSW noted that their reflection had been emotional as well as rational. There has been a sense that NQSWs were able to understand their critical incident better and think about it in a helpful manner that leads to practising in a clearer way with less confusion or conflicting emotions. One NQSW noted that they felt meeting for critical reflection groups outside their office space had been valuable, as they felt this provided a more objective or neutral environment in which to be able to reflect.

NQSWs have spoken about the fact that critical reflection has enabled them to reflect on their assumptions and how these impact on their practice. This has also been linked to workers reflecting that they feel more self-aware and have developed a greater understanding of colleagues, which has led to a more meaningful understanding of their team and how it can function. Fook and Gardner (2007) similarly recognise that one of the benefits and outcomes of critical reflection is that practitioners accept integration of personal and professional experiences.

When cases become confused and messy, we can sometimes struggle to see a way forward or imagine the situation changing, as we can become enmeshed within the problem and the anxieties this can bring. By becoming 'unstuck' and being able to find ways of progressing through a difficult issue, practitioners are more easily able to think about the issue. This has resulted in NQSWs feeling more confident and emotionally safe to think about complex cases in a stable and rational manner. This is in line with Fook and Gardner's (2007) recognition that critical reflection can help participants feel 'empowered' by the process. This is seen when workers move from feeling stuck to feeling 'unstuck' and able to see new ways of practising, which Fook and Gardner (2007) list as another benefit of critical reflection.

What has stood out significantly whilst facilitating critical reflection group sessions has been the value that professionals, irrelevant of experience, place on being listened to. The fact that the group process does not set out to affirm actions or thinking of participants was not a hindrance to workers feeling supported simply by being listened to. This reflects Donnellan and Jack's (2010: 134) view that NQSWs need to have a safe place in which to discuss their work and find release for their emotional responses to it. Donnellan and Jack (2010: 134) also discuss the importance of NQSWs feeling they have 'permission' to express angry feelings, and refer to evidence by Bednar (2003) to suggest that there is a negative effect on outcomes for service users where anger remains 'cooped up' inside.

Future directions

In order to address attendance issues, we have created two more critical reflection groups, which will ensure the sessions are area-based and close to the social workers who need to attend. This also means that smaller groups can be run, which can contribute to participants getting to know one another better and developing a more cohesive group dynamic. I have learned that making sessions accessible is of importance to NQSWs so that they cut down on travel time. It is, however, still important to make sure the sessions are in a private venue that can ensure confidentiality and no interruption.

A further practical change has been to book dates of sessions with further notice and to ensure that NQSWs' line managers are aware of the sessions in order to encourage their support for NQSWs to attend, as well as arranging schedules to support their availability. I feel this has raised the profile of the critical reflection sessions, and NQSWs are feeling more able to prioritise attending critical reflection sessions with the support of their manager. This support is particularly important for NQSWs and helps them say 'no' when they need to in order to prioritise attending their critical reflection session.

Currently, critical reflection sessions are being run just with NQSWs and the supervising RSWs at the residential home. Considering the interest shown by other experienced social workers and managers, I hope that in the future we will be able to make these sessions available to more staff. I feel there is great value in the critical reflection process, and believe that being able to critically reflect on practice is integral to our learning and development. Munro (2011) states that intuitive and analytical reasoning skills are developed in different ways, and talks about the need for child protection services to recognise the differing requirements if practitioners are to develop from novices to experts in both intuitive and analytical reasoning skills. She also goes on to say that intuitive skills are essentially derived from experience, but experience on its own is not enough – it needs to be 'allied to reflection – time and attention given to mulling over the experience and learning from it'. A group form of critical reflection could be a significant medium through which social care staff can develop this expertise. Munro (2011) also acknowledges that time and critical reflection in supervision is needed in order to apply the range of knowledge, skills and values required to carry out effective social work. Using the Fook/Gardner 2007 model for critical reflection within group supervision may provide a valuable format in which to ensure critical reflection within supervision and drive forward this important recommendation.

References

Bednar, S.G. (2003) 'Elements of satisfying organisational climates in child welfare agencies', *Families in Society*, 84: 7–12.

Donnellan, H. and Jack, G. (2010) *The Survival Guide for Newly Qualified Child and Family Social Workers*, London: Jessica Kingsley.

Fook, J. and Gardner, F. (2007) *Practising Critical Reflection: A Resource Handbook*, Maidenhead: Open University Press.

Howe, D. (2009) *A Brief Introduction to Social Work Theory*, Houndmills: Palgrave Macmillan.

Jackson, M. (2007) *The Post-Qualifying Handbook for Social Workers*, London: Jessica Kingsley.

Lawson, H. (2002) *The Blackwell Companion to Social Work*, Oxford: Blackwell Publishing.

Munro, E. (2011) *The Munro Review of Child Protection: Final Report – A Child-centred System*, Norwich: The Stationery Office.

8 Critical reflection and supervision

An interdisciplinary experience

Fiona Gardner and Eddie Taalman[1]

Health professionals generally work in interdisciplinary teams and are expected to manage the complexities of engaging with those from differing professional backgrounds. Critical reflection based on Fook and Gardner (2007) can provide a language and framework for working across disciplines. This chapter outlines the experience of an interdisciplinary team in a health service – the Rehabilitation in the Home team (RITH) at Southern Health – in implementing peer supervision groups using critical reflection. Rehabilitation in the home is a home-based program providing intensive rehabilitation services to the Southern Metropolitan region in Victoria, Australia, with offices located at three different nodes across the region. Unlike many of the other existing home-based rehabilitation programs, Southern Health RITH provides both case management and Allied Health therapy from the following disciplines: speech therapy, dietetics, neuropsychology, occupational therapy, physiotherapy and social work. The current RITH case managers are all qualified professionals from a variety of backgrounds, including occupational therapy, social work and nursing. This provides a wide variety of educational backgrounds and varied theoretical knowledge bases, but also poses a unique challenge for peer supervision using critical reflection. The disciplines felt safe within the context of their own discipline, but then had to meet the challenge of working across disciplines.

Southern Health is a large metropolitan health service with 400 professionals in its Allied Health Continuing Care Program (full- and part-time). In 2007, Allied Health began a supervision project aiming to implement supervision practice in the Continuing Care Program, and my co-author (Eddie Taalman) was seconded as a .4 EFT project manager. A panel of senior clinical staff and discipline-based managers, along with the Allied Health Director and Eddie as project manager, was established to provide input into drafting supervision guidelines for the nine professional groupings: physiotherapy, occupational therapy, speech pathology, social work, psychology, dietetics, podiatry, music therapy and exercise physiology. At that stage, clinical supervision varied significantly across disciplines and service areas, with some having established supervision practices and others with no formalised supervision system in place.

The next stage of the project was to enlist the support of line and discipline managers, in late February 2008. They were briefed about the supervision guidelines and consulted about the issues and challenges of supervision. According to Rolfe:

> Definitions of clinical supervision abound; put simply, clinical supervision can be described as a flexible and dynamic structure within which to continuously deconstruct and reconstruct clinical practice. Fundamental to this process of deconstruction and reconstruction are the skills of reflection, critical reflection and reflexivity. In other words, clinical supervision and reflective practice are interdependent and inextricably linked through the process of reflection.
>
> (Rolfe, 2011b: 103)

It was agreed to pursue a reflective model of supervision that would ideally be used in peer supervision groups.

At this time, I was offering training in supervision and critical reflection through the Centre for Professional Development at Latrobe University. The Allied Health Director and Eddie as supervision project manager agreed on six two-day training programs over the following eighteen months, and six half-day follow-up sessions. Critical reflection was considered to offer a

> broad analytical approach to exploring matters that arise for the individual in the clinical setting. Its aim is to encourage active learning, through thinking and talking about particular issues that impact and affect the individual. The relationship is collegiate in nature, offering all parties the opportunity to learn and develop during the supervision process.
>
> (Taalman, 2009: 4)

The training included a general introduction to supervision principles and practices, with a particular focus on the Fook and Gardner (2007) model of critical reflection. The first day began by exploring current issues for professional practice, and related these to the kinds of issues likely to arise in supervision. Different supervision definitions and models were identified (Kadushin, 1985; Proctor, 2001), and how supervision has changed over time was discussed, with questioning of the more traditional one-to-one approach and more interest in group supervision (Cutliffe et al., 2001). Exploring contemporary thinking about supervision included the use of critical reflection as well as peer and group supervision (Hawkins and Shohet, 2006).

The second day of training began by identifying and discussing the underlying theory of critical reflection used by Fook and Gardner (2007), followed by explaining the critical reflection process. We then discussed the 'culture of acceptance' in critical reflection, before working with an experience of mine over stages one and two. Participants then divided into groups of three and took it in turns to explore an experience of their own. The timing of this was managed so that each participant had specific amounts of time for stages one and two and debriefing, before going on to the next person. I was explicit that these times were more artificial than would necessarily happen in a supervision group, but that I wanted everyone to have at least a beginning experience of using the process. Given the pressure in health care to find solutions, this also ensured that participants spent sufficient time on stage one to explore the experience. Having groups of three also allowed participants some idea of how this might work in a supervision group, while being small enough not to be daunting. We then debriefed as a whole group, identifying both what was useful to notice about the process (what worked), and questions and issues raised, which we discussed. Helpful questions were noted, adding these to the list generated from my example. After the training, participants were assigned to multidisciplinary supervision groups, which could also include staff who had not completed training.

Follow-up sessions were held with each of the training groups approximately six to twelve months later. These sessions began with feedback about how individuals and groups were using the ideas and processes discussed in training, and comments about how they would like to use this session. All the groups requested more practice with critical reflection, so in each session a participant volunteered an experience and we worked as a whole group with their example. Feedback suggested that this was helpful in consolidating understanding of the process.

This chapter focuses on the experience of one team at Southern Health: the Rehabilitation in the Home team (RITH). Senior staff at RITH had two aims in establishing the critical reflection model in their supervision groups: actively to support uptake of the training provided; and also to build interdisciplinary teamwork and the connections between teams at different sites. Because of this, they allocated people to groups, trying to balance teams' professional background and experience with the critical reflection model. All staff were expected to participate in the process initially. The RITH management also asked me to attend each supervision group in 2010 for whatever the particular group suggested would be useful for them. Generally, I participated in the group either as a facilitator or group member, having a discussion with each group towards the end of the session about what was working well and any issues or dilemmas raised.

In 2011, I met with Eddie initially, then with the RITH manager and coordinator to explore following up the supervision groups as part of writing this chapter about the experience at Southern Health. Partly because of my previous attendance at the groups, I suggested that I would offer to attend another session of each group before meeting with any group members interested in an evaluation focus group. However, the ethics committee at Southern Health felt that we needed an independent person to run the focus groups. In the end, I attended a session of four supervision groups, and Jill Hanlon, a colleague experienced in running critical reflection groups, facilitated the focus group sessions immediately afterwards. A fifth group chose not to participate. One person from this group chose to be interviewed on his own. The focus groups were entirely voluntary and were attended by a total of twenty participants. The focus group questions were grouped into several areas as follows:

- In retrospect, what was useful about the training and what would you recommend be done differently?
- What do you see as the benefits of and barriers to this form of peer supervision?
- What has helped this process (critical reflection and group supervision) to work?
- What difference, if any, does this make to your practice?
- What are the challenges to using the critical reflection approach in your work practice? (for example, the way you work with clients and your general approach to work).

Training

Participants who had experienced it were generally positive about the training, particularly the practice of critical reflection and having follow-up sessions to consolidate learning once they had had a chance to practise on their own. Having a facilitator experienced in the process was helpful. Accessible language and examples made the underlying theory more understandable, though still daunting to some. They also appreciated the organisation offering such training, though some would have liked greater clarity about who could access it, and why, and the purpose of the supervision groups.

Benefits

A consistent, significant benefit was learning and consolidating the critical reflection process of exploring a particular experience more deeply and becoming able to identify underlying assumptions. Having the two stages of critical reflection meant that participants could feel free to explore and understand their experience at a significantly deeper level without the pressure of seeking a solution. Knowing this was available helped some: 'if I've got an issue I know I've got a forum to discuss it in before I maybe take it elsewhere'. Participants also frequently identified the value of hearing that other people's issues and assumptions were very similar to theirs. As one said, 'I think it, the universal issue, which is about reflection is ... you feel better about yourself in a way because sometimes you internalise or personalise the issues and you realise that they are universal and everyone's got the same issues.' Related to this, another saw critical reflection as a 'power-sharing process' different from the usual medical model.

There was universal agreement about the benefit of having interdisciplinary teams, though some participants had felt unsure about this in the beginning.

Group members understood more fully the challenges and perspectives important to other disciplines. This was seen as having several benefits: first, it often became clear that issues were shared across disciplines, which increased participants' comfort in working with each other. At the same time, participants appreciated the differences that different disciplines brought and the new perceptions they gained about a particular situation.

A related benefit was that the process of critical reflection helped build a sense of team or group trust, enabling participants to get to know each other more deeply and to feel a greater sense of mutual support and trust from others in their critical reflection group. Expressing themselves freely in a mutually supportive setting was particularly valued by most participants, including being able to name and explore emotions as needed, and having a forum to 'name difficult things'. For many participants, this meant they felt more able to seek help and support from others in their particular group, outside the sessions. It also meant that if there was some kind of conflict with those in their group, including from a clinical perspective, participants were more confident about being able to discuss and resolve this . For example, one critical reflection was: 'Particularly helpful in resolving a conflict I was having within the organisation. This was a real "ah-ha" moment.'

Participants suggested that critically reflecting in their group helped them learn from each other about how to handle different situations, gaining ideas from other people's assumptions, feelings, thoughts and actions, as well as strategies that emerged from the process. As one said, 'I feel that I got to benefit from other people's experiences so that I can apply them to relevant experiences in my role.' Participants also valued having both genders represented in groups, another different perspective.

Barriers and dilemmas

One of the most consistently identified barriers was changing group membership as staff left, changed roles or went on maternity leave. Having new people arrive in the group was experienced as problematic, partly because of the challenge of orienting new participants who had not always completed training, and partly because it disrupted the established sense of trust and group culture. Some groups had found ways to manage this, particularly if there was still a core of skilled and committed participants who could then familiarise new members. How new people were oriented varied: some had managed to do some training; others hadn't. Some had read the written material accompanying training which helped; but others felt it was only after attending training or seeing how the group worked over time that they gained understanding of the process. Two participants felt they never really had.

This relates to the second consistent finding: the difficulty of engaging people who are simply not interested in this approach or find it too confronting or too personal. For some, this connected to the barrier of not having been able to participate in training. As one person pointed out, having even one negative person can mean that others are not prepared to be as open. This raises questions about who decides who is in the group, how people are allocated, and how to balance personalities, disciplines and sites. It was felt to be better for management to continue to do this and to be the point of contact where participation was not working. A potential barrier here was people feeling that some disciplines, such as social workers, had more experience of reflection built into their professional training and practice.

Two of the groups thought a lack of clarity about some aspects of the group could be an actual or potential barrier. These included transparency about whether participation was voluntary, and the need for all participants to be clear about the purpose of the supervision groups and that they are supported by management. This could help with another barrier expressed by some: the tension between prioritising other work, particularly client work, and the supervision group. As one person said, 'a lot of times with supervision and critical reflection there comes a time when the rest of your load is running at almost capacity and I don't know if the expectations from your supervisor or immediate heads, where do you put your priority?'. This compares with others who felt, for example, 'you have to give yourself permission to go. This is for me, I'm going.'

This connects to the next barrier: time combined with the complications of getting everyone together, often across different sites. While people valued having the mixture in the group, this did create another time pressure, given that some participants had to travel. Time also created a dilemma when a particular incident raised issues for others in the group that there wasn't time to engage with, generally because people had other commitments. One group identified this as an issue for which they needed a strategy. Finally, several mentioned the difficulty of thinking of an appropriate incident, although others suggested that once the group started, ideas soon emerged.

What helped the process?

Implicit in much of what participants explored in the focus groups was what helped the supervision groups to work well. All the groups agreed that it was important to make the group a priority, to be committed to the process, and also to frequent and regular sessions (usually every six weeks). This provided the means to consolidate learning from the training by practising the process. Ideally, it was felt that the groups needed to be established soon after training for this reason.

Participants acknowledged that the groups, like any groups, have periods when they work better than others, partly with new people joining and those with established critical reflection skills leaving. Sometimes this meant the group felt it needed to start by building the group culture again; perhaps stopping the critical reflection process and getting to know each other first. While the need for this had been acknowledged in the training, for some this felt frustrating. As one participant said 'you kind of get on a roll and things start, you get a bit more confident in the questions you are asking, but when you have time away, you have to learn it again and you lose the momentum'. For others this was simply an inevitable part of the group work process, 'when the group was first set up the idea was to get people to just have a bit of a social thing, some of them here, they went and had a coffee together so that was non-threatening, and next time was, let's start doing something'.

Most of the groups also identified the importance of having individuals take on particular roles, particularly the role of facilitator to maintain focus and the use of agreed group culture. Generally this role, and roles such as timekeeper or writer on the whiteboard, were rotated. This also helped to ensure the group planned ahead, having people volunteer to present in the following session/s. One group had a roster for the year, with some flexibility built in for anything urgent. Most of the groups had an expectation that everyone would take a turn to present so that 'everyone's views would be represented' and/or because this encouraged a sense of mutual trust in the group. Groups identified specific tools that helped, such as the material that came with training (articles and notes), the use of a whiteboard, writing up the experience to be presented, using brainstorming, and a set of examples of questions that had been developed after the training. Two groups had initially developed an agreement about group process, which had also been helpful in building trust and clarifying expectations.

It was also seen as helpful to make sure everybody had received the initial training and a refresher or follow-up session at some point after that – one group suggested three months later, another six months. Those who had received the follow-up session that connected to the initial training felt this had been an important point in consolidating their learning. Finally, having flexibility to decide on the time and place of the group was identified as helpful.

Influence on practice

Becoming more reflective was identified as the main influence on practice, particularly in terms of exploring experiences and questioning assumptions. As one participant said: 'I don't think it's my natural personality because I'm a problem solver ... so bringing it back and examining it all and doing the assumptions doesn't come naturally, but it's really beneficial.' In all the groups, some people identified changed thinking about what they had assumed about themselves and also about others. Developing this capacity enabled participants to look more deeply into the underlying causes of particular reactions, to 'think what might be going on for them, their assumptions'. This was seen as particularly helpful in working with complex behaviour or situations. For some, this was displayed in changed thinking and developing the capacity to see a situation from other perspectives, as suggested in this interaction:

'Increased awareness, not making judgements.

Even though it is an obvious question about assumptions – what is it that we are assuming and the other people who are involved assuming? – sometimes that delves a little deeper into what is going on.

It does just prompt you to step into other people's shoes, whether it be other people in the group, like the presenter, or the situation they are presenting about.'

This process of exploring assumptions led to the value of taking a step back, not just having 'knee-jerk reactions', or 'pulling things apart rather than just fix it'. The process of identifying what was happening at a deeper level sometimes led to better solutions, or at other times clarified that it wasn't possible to 'fix' the situation, but that it was possible to see all sides. Some identified this as influencing them to ask why, rather than giving an answer or specific suggestions to another professional, or at least not immediately: 'so I think we come up with solutions because we are able to talk around things, reflect on it first. And I find it's more satisfying.' Others identified the value of asking open and open-ended questions.

All groups identified the value of the process for illustrating the variety of ways in which one might respond to a particular situation. The multiplicity of disciplines and backgrounds helped generate a diversity of ideas. Even when working with somebody else's example, participants felt they could make connections to their own experiences and generate ideas about what might be possible for them. Individuals also identified specific changes in attitude, such as 'the ability to say no and reflecting on that, and what that means to me as a professional, and how I go about it in an ethical way'. Changed reactions to clients included: 'I think the training changed how I ask clients questions as well and encourage their reflection'; and, from another, being 'conscious of sometimes I'm actually trying to push them somewhere without actually trying to listen … I think it just gives … The space to think about it … Its a choice about whether you want to do it one way or another.'

A particular change in practice was changed attitudes to other disciplines in general, as well as more specifically to those in the critical reflection group. This partly came from seeing that other disciplines experience similar feelings and challenges, and thus feeling less 'threatened' by them. The experience of belonging in the supervision group generally meant developing 'respect and rapport' for and with other disciplines. More specifically, participants felt they knew each other's feelings, reactions and thought processes at a deeper level. They had also developed a sense of openness to difference as part of the group, which made it easier to approach others about complex or difficult issues in the workplace. Because of this attitude some participants felt more empowered or confident in raising issues of conflict, particularly with those in the group, but for some at least, also with others from outside the group. This seemed to relate back to attitudes about diversity, being able to see that people could perceive and experience the same things quite differently. As one said, it 'is that people work differently and in this group setting you can actually address that and it's an acceptance and you can be quite relaxed if it happened outside of this setting'.

Participants in two groups made an important distinction between what they did in the supervision groups as part of a critically reflective process, and what they did in case management or case discussions, perhaps because of the pressures of time there to achieve specific clinical outcomes. In critical reflection, what they were doing was exploring their general approach to work rather than discipline-related strategies about treating a specific illness or condition. One person, for example, said 'it's not so much about how a physio does their work, or a nurse does their work, or how I do my work, maybe it's how I might respond to somebody, because we have discussed things to take into account personal and professional relationships and what that means. And just listening to the themes that arise you find is a commonality between the whole lot of us.' Another group did include reflection on what they saw as clinical issues, but made a similar distinction: 'it's usually about how you manage complex behaviours, not so much your actual therapy intervention, it's how you're dealing with a difficult person and how you're maintaining a positive approach'.

One group particularly felt it was interesting that the attitudes of critical reflection, the different ways of listening and questioning, hadn't transferred over to case management discussions in the organisation. However, groups did consider organisational issues related to their experiences. Two groups had also used the critical reflection process to reflect more deeply on particular organisational change. Some in supervisory positions were using critical reflection as part of supervision.

Future directions

The findings from this research affirm the value of critical reflection supervision groups across disciplines for deepening joint exploration of complex practice issues and increasing the capacity of those from different disciplines to work effectively together. Many of the benefits reinforce the outcomes identified by Fook and Gardner (2007): an increased sense of connectedness to others in the team; a validation of the place of emotion; seeing new possibilities for perceiving what was happening as well as for changed actions, which was often empowering. This is supported by the experience of Fronek et al. (2009: 26), who provided training using critical reflection across health, welfare and education disciplines, and found that 'Participants reported positive benefits of sharing knowledge and experiences with practitioners from other disciplinary groups.' They recommended that 'A supervision model suitable for interdisciplinary teams needs consideration.'

The value of learning from experience as part of the critical reflection approach is also reinforced by the findings. Boud and Garrick (1999: 8) suggest that 'Experience is the foundation of, and the stimulus for, learning.' From their experience of providing continuing education to a group of occupational therapists, Vachon et al. (2010: 345) recommended that future programs 'promote the development of their reflective skills by supporting the sharing of authentic and personal experiences'. Participants at RITH implied that the value of this may come partly from naming and engaging with the emotions generated from such experiences, which is again supported by Vachon et al., as well as Huffington et al. (2004), in exploring the impact of organisational life.

Many participants were also able to identify change in their practice in using the model: some individual changes in relation to client work, or in attitudes and values. More consistently, there were changed attitudes to those from other disciplines and to confidence in raising potentially difficult issues with others. The two stages of the critical reflection model were important in generating change: first in understanding an experience more deeply, articulating assumptions and seeing different perspectives; then identifying possible strategies and 'solutions' helped with changed action. This is reinforced by the experience of Vachon et al. (2010: 344) who found that reflection alone did not bring about change unless there were recommendations for action in practice.

What helped the process is also clear: shared training experiences, clarity from the organisation about the aims of supervision groups and expectations of participation. Having a facilitator was seen as important both for the initial training and for the supervision groups to work well. Rolfe (2011a: 137) suggests 'The dangers of unfacilitated groups cannot be overstated' in ensuring that groups maintain focus and a positive group culture. While he advocates that, for some situations, a skilled and experienced facilitator is needed, for others he simply means that the role is important in the group. The facilitator was also important in guiding the group's process and proposing different strategies to improve participants' reflective learning skills.

The training at Southern Health also included a brief session on group processes, at the request of the project manager. This included the importance of building trust and group culture, and possible challenges of group dynamics. There can be a tendency in setting up critical reflection or other supervision groups to assume that professionals already have such knowledge. The experience here reinforces how this can help manage the inevitable changes in groups. Related to this is the value of management, as was the case here, recognising and validating the time taken to build the group culture.

The findings here raise the question of whether critical reflection in peer supervision is for everyone. What isn't totally clear is how much of the value was in critical reflection and how much in being in a group, particularly where the group was more experienced in the process than new individual members. Todd (2005) questions how effective reflective practice is for practitioners who are defensive about their practice, so only bring 'success cases' to supervision. She suggests that some people need what she calls 'life supervision', working on specific, concrete activities and discussing them. Similarly,

Vachon et al. (2010: 340) found that some participants 'were more conservative and did not spontaneously try to apply the new knowledge in their practice. Their perspective changes remained untested and, by the end of the study, were not yet integrated into their personal practice theory.' There may be something inherently contradictory in expecting critical reflection to suit everyone, given its underlying valuing of diversity. It would certainly be useful to explore what individuals find challenging about the process in supervision groups to clarify the issues. It may well be that for some people, generally or at particular times, other forms of supervision are more appropriate.

The findings also suggest the challenges of embedding critical reflection attitudes throughout organisational practices. One group had used supervision sessions to reflect collectively on organisational change, and all the groups referred to common themes related to organisational issues. Some participants were puzzled that the critically reflective attitudes that were so helpful in their supervision groups were not used in other, more clinically oriented case discussion groups. As other participants suggested, this may be related to the pressures of time for clinical outcomes. However, it does suggest the value of having opportunities such as this, perhaps facilitated, to reflect on the critical reflection process and its impact on practice and the potential for organisational change.

Note

1 Acknowledgement: we would particularly like to acknowledge the contributions of all those who came to the focus groups or were interviewed individually, as well as Andrea Williams and Siobhan McGinness, who provided significant support in enabling the focus groups to happen and in commenting on the draft of this chapter.

References

Boud, D. and Garrick, J. (eds) (1999) *Understanding Learning at Work*, London: Routledge.

Cutliffe, J.R., Butterworth, T. and Proctor, B. (eds) (2001) *20 Fundamental Themes in Supervision*, London: Routledge.

Fook, J. and Gardner, F. (2007) *Practising Critical Reflection: A Resource Handbook*, Maidenhead: Open University Press.

Fronek, P., Kendall, M., Ungerer, G., Malt, A., Eugarde, E.A. and Geraghty, T. (2009) 'Towards healthy professional–client relationships: the value of an interprofessional training course', *Journal of Interprofessional Care*, 23(1): 16–19.

Hawkins, P. and Shohet, R. (2006) *Supervision in the Helping Professions* (3rd edn), Maidenhead: McGraw Hill/Open University Press.

Huffington, C., Armstrong, D., Halton, W., Hoyle, L.A. and Pooley, J. (2004) *Working Below the Surface: The Emotional Life of Contemporary Organizations*, London: Karnac.

Kadushin, A. (1985) *Supervision in Social Work*, New York: Columbia University Press.

Proctor, B. (2001) 'Training for the supervision alliance: attitude, skills and intention', in Cutliffe, J.R., Butterworth, T. and Proctor, B. (eds), *20 Fundamental Themes in Supervision*, London: Routledge.

Rolfe, G. (2011a) 'Group supervision', in Rolfe, G., Jasper, M. and Freshwater, D. (eds), *Critical Reflection in Practice: Generating Knowledge for Care*, Houndmills: Palgrave Macmillan, 127–59.

——(2011b) 'Clinical supervision and reflective practice', in Rolfe, G., Jasper, M. and Freshwater, D. (eds), *Critical Reflection in Practice: Generating Knowledge for Care*, Houndmills: Palgrave Macmillan, 100–26.

Taalman, E. (2009) 'The Application of Supervision across Allied Health within the Continuing Care Program – Southern Health', 2007–9 Program Implementation Project Report, Clayton: Southern Health.

Todd, G. (2005) 'Reflective practice and Socratic dialogue', in Johns, C. and Freshwater, D. (eds), *Transforming Nursing Through Reflective Practice* (2nd edn), Oxford: Blackwell Publishing, 38–54.

Vachon, B., Durand, M.-J. and LeBlanc, J. (2010) 'Using reflective learning to improve the impact of continuing education in the context of work rehabilitation', *Advances in Health Sciences Education*, 15(3): 329–48.

9 Thinking critically about student supervision

Lynne Allan

Introduction

Learning critical reflection skills can be highly valuable for students undertaking field placements in health and welfare agencies. Whilst providing theoretical frameworks to inform their practice, critical reflection also develops students' ability to critically examine their own practice and therefore the impact this has on their work with clients. This is particularly important given increasing complexities and uncertainty in the organisational contexts that practitioners face in everyday work in the human services sector, including an expectation of multidisciplinary practice. This chapter examines the value of group supervision to teach critical reflection skills for social work and welfare students completing student field placements in a large government organisation in Victoria, Australia. The supervision uses the Fook/Gardner critical reflection model, and was developed from observations and experience of the potential benefits for students and the model's applicability across a range of disciplines.

I first developed an interest in critical reflection in 2004 after attending a two-day critical reflection introductory training workshop, facilitated by Fiona Gardner, using the Fook/Gardner model of critical reflection. In this training, I discovered that critical reflection offered a model which went beyond the 'traditional' reflection I was familiar with. I found it was a model with which I could examine and reflect on my practice in environments characterised by change, uncertainty and complexity, which I felt was more useful in current practice and organisational contexts. This was reinforced by attending more advanced training about using the model in supervision and research, facilitated by either Jan Fook or Fiona Gardner. I felt so inspired by this model, and what it offered to me and my practice as a social worker, that I wanted other workers, particularly students, to be given the opportunity to learn about critical reflection. I was aware, through my own studies and organisational role coordinating student placements, that 'reflective practice' was a focus in universities and tertiary institutions in their social work and welfare-related courses; however, critical reflection appeared to be seen as fairly new. I knew from my own learning about critical reflection that it wasn't something you could just read about in a book; rather it was a process you needed to learn and experience to gain a good understanding of how to use it to examine your own practice. Fook (2008: vi) suggests that 'Critical reflection can challenge mainstream intellectual culture which underpins professional practice, therefore it needs to be explicitly taught and learnt in order to maximise a particular type of learning.'

Within my organisation, we had a structure in place for students on placement, which included group peer supervision. This occurred on a monthly basis, and was mainly for mutual support and feedback about placement progress and any issues requiring discussion. I decided that the monthly group peer supervision provided a structure that I could expand to incorporate critical reflection. Hawkins and Shohet (2000: 23, 128) suggest that supervision is a central form of support for workers in organisations, providing a safe setting in which workers can reflect on and learn from difficulties, including emotions that they may be experiencing. It can give workers the opportunity to stand back and reflect, and provide an opportunity to find new alternatives. This can be enhanced in a group setting where the group provides peer support, opportunities for identification of shared experiences and feedback, reflections and input from colleagues.

The Fook/Gardner critical reflection model appealed to me, as I liked the structure and process used and the theoretical frameworks that underpinned it. I felt these were essential for students to enable them to analyse and develop their practice and to critically examine practice contexts. The students who came on placement in my organisation were predominantly social workers or in welfare-related disciplines, but I was also aware that we sometimes had students on placement from other disciplines, such as nursing and speech pathology. My observations from the Fook/Gardner critical reflection training workshops was that participants were from a range of organisations and backgrounds, which led me to believe that the model could be multidisciplinary and fit well within my organisational context. This was confirmed for me after running the group sessions, and reflected in the evaluations of students.

> 'I found critical reflection very useful and relevant no matter what program area we were in, what field we wanted to go into after finishing university or what year of study we were in.'

Given that critical reflection was not well known, I decided to call the group supervision model 'reflective practice sessions' at first, as I felt that this was a known practice process and so would address any barriers to participation that the term 'critical reflection' might evoke. I made this decision as I had found that sometimes people thought I meant to 'criticise' practice, which may have deterred students from participating, or influenced supervisors' support of student participation. At a later date, when critical reflection became more well known and understood, I was able to call the group supervision 'critical reflection'.

> During implementation of the critical reflection model, I began studying a Master's course based around critical reflection, so as I was implementing the model into my organisation, I was also continuing to learn about critical reflection. I conducted evaluations from each group of students and used these to inform and shape the model and therefore critically reflect on my own practice.

Implementing critical reflection for student supervision

The model of critical reflection I used followed fairly closely the Fook/Gardner model and underpinning theories because of its ability to be adapted to a range of contexts and disciplines. The groups consisted of eight to ten students from a mixture of disciplines. Frequency of sessions depended on the length of placements, but was usually a three-hour session four times in a fourteen-week placement, approximately four weeks apart. Information about the groups was sent to students beforehand and, whilst the expectation was that all students would participate in the group, participation was voluntary, as was the presentation of an incident.

Session one

The first session was similar to that of the Fook/Gardner model and aimed to create a safe environment. Specifically, the tasks were as follows:

1. Set agreed group guidelines/rules for session to create a safe environment. Students always put forward rules around respect, confidentiality, being non-judgemental and listening to others' opinions.
2. Introduce critical reflection and the underpinning theoretical frameworks of critical social theory, postmodernism, poststructuralism, reflective practice, reflexivity and deconstruction. I use a range of adult learning tools to assist with this, using a teaching type of format. This includes handouts about critical reflection with information about the Fook/Gardner Model and process. I use an interactive style and focus particularly on students gaining a good understanding of 'binary language' and the impact this can have on categorisation and power relations. I have found that this session is the most important as it lays the foundations for the rest of the process, provides the theoretical 'lens' through which students are able to examine their assumptions and incident, and challenges students to begin to think outside of the mainstream.
3. Introduce and explain the Fook/Gardner two-stage critical reflection model and process.

4. Explain the questioning involved in the process to assist presenters, and explain my role in guiding them in those questions – that the aim is to help the person unpack their incident and their thinking around this, and that the group's role is to assist them in this, but not to make judgements around what they did or impose our own views around what they did through our questions.

5. Present my own critical reflection incident to demonstrate the critical reflection process of the Fook/Gardner two-stage model. The incident I use is a personal incident that demonstrates to the group my preparedness to be vulnerable, to participate in a critical reflection process and to examine my assumptions on a personal level. This also demonstrates how the personal and professional are inextricably linked together, and how critical reflection reveals/unearths this. In this sense, it demonstrates that it does not matter if the incident they choose is a professional or personal one.

6. Explain that presentation is voluntary. Students are given a choice as to whether they make a presentation. Whilst students can sometimes express feeling anxious about presenting, presenting my own critical reflection incident seems to assist in allaying their anxiety, and I have not had any student present an incident who said afterwards they wished they hadn't. Rather, students comment that they were really happy they had decided to present an incident.

Sessions two to four

These sessions consisted of student presentations, aiming for approximately one hour per student.

The model used thus did not differ significantly from the Fook/Gardner model, except that it was conducted over a period of 3.5 months, and that both stages happened within one session.

Emerging assumptions

The first set of assumptions relate to the complexity of practice and the organisational context. Students had often previously made assumptions about the clarity and certainty of professional practice. From their own and shared experiences, they developed new assumptions related to the uncertainty and complexity of organisational and practice environments. They shifted to some degree from expecting that they could predict practice and always provide definite answers and predict definite directions, to assumptions that the direction may not be clear and that the ideal may not be possible given organisational resources and expectations.

New assumptions also developed in relation to the connections between personal and professional; theory and practice. Previously, students had tended to see these as binaries, an either/or. Their assumptions changed to understand how these ideally are seen as connected. This related to a previous assumption about setting aside their own values and reactions to a new assumption about the need for awareness, and constructive use of these. Specifically, students developed new assumptions about the influence their personal values had on their practice, and ultimately on clients, leading to a more reflexive view of practice.

The shared experiences in the group also changed assumptions about the individual nature of experience to seeing that experiences were shared and had structural underpinnings. New assumptions included that this is a general issue; this is not just about me. Power was seen as more complex and something that could be enacted more than previously thought.

The second set of assumptions related to the need for continuing to include and integrate critical reflection into future practice and supervision, due to the benefits it provided both personally and professionally, and for clients. Previously, this was not something that most students had considered, but their new assumption was that this would be an important aspect of effective practice.

My own observations and reflections

Linking theory to practice/making meaning

I found that often students were not familiar with theories such as post-modernism, or if they had learned about them in their studies, they did not make links between these theories and practice. Therefore the session that introduces these theories is important in assisting them not only to understand the theories underpinning critical reflection, but also to be able to make links to practice. The theoretical framework with which the students seem to connect most strongly is the dichotomous thinking/language and binary constructions, as they are able to locate this within their own experiences, and from this identify how it links to power and power relationships, marginalisation, social and political structures, and the allocation and distribution of resources. It appears that binary constructions provide the framework or link which students use to make sense or meaning of critical reflection, which was a new experience for a large number of students (Mezirow and Associates, 2000: 16, 114).

Challenges and barriers

Students commented on the strong emotions which their presentation and the process could evoke within them and other presenters. Fook and Askeland (2006) highlight that 'participants in critical reflection can sometimes express a desire to "protect" others from strong feelings and the risk of challenge which might be evoked during the critical reflection process. Despite this they state that participants report a transformative experience from their participation in the critical reflection process.' This view was reflected by students who said that they found presenting an incident very challenging and exposing of themselves and their values and assumptions. However, they felt they gained much from their participation in the process. For this reason, they felt that participation/attendance at the sessions should be compulsory and given a priority within their placement. This comment came from a group where some students had not attended all sessions as placement work tasks had been given priority over attendance.

Non-attendance may indicate a view that reflecting on practice is not seen to be as important as work tasks by students or supervisors; or a reluctance by students to participate due to apprehension about the process, a lack of understanding of critical reflection or a fear of their practice being scrutinised. This further highlights the importance of a safe environment, particularly given that students are being assessed for competence in their placement. By participating, students are putting their practice up for scrutiny, so a high level of safety to do that is important.

Critical reflection is not a concept or process that everyone finds useful for examining their practice, as it challenges us to examine ourselves and our own values and assumptions, which not all practitioners may be willing to do. Some participants grappled with the concept of the link between the personal and professional, feeling that some presentations were 'too personal'. This could also reflect an espoused view which exists within some welfare and health sectors that the personal and professional should remain separate. Not all students who participated in the critical reflection process grasped the concept of reflexivity. Some tended to want to place 'blame' on other people within their presented scenario, rather than exploring how their own assumptions and values had informed or influenced their practice within their presented incident.

Students also found developing and using appropriate questions challenging. Even though I provided guidance throughout the process, and gave guidelines and examples of critical questions in the first session, students often struggled with asking a question to the presenting person that was not imposing their own ideas/values and judgements. Students commented that their participation assisted them to be able to learn how to ask questions, which helped people to unpack their own thinking rather than the person asking the question imposing theirs. This further highlights that the facilitator and their role is critical to the process.

Facilitators must have the ability to ask critical questions, or facilitate the group asking critical questions, that will elicit assumptions, beliefs and values. This takes a high level of skill, and at times I found it difficult to guide the questions from other group participants without appearing to be judgemental of them, which could be a contradictory to the process and the guidelines set by the group. Brookfield (1987: 90–95) supports the view that 'role modeling of the process and theoretical frameworks appears to be an important part of the critical reflection process … that is facilitators have to be congruent with the theories and process being espoused and demonstrate a preparedness to be open to take risks and analyse their own assumptions'. Presenting my own critical incident, I believe, assists in achieving this, developing trust within the group and trust of the facilitator. Brookfield (1987: 91–95) asserts that facilitators must earn trust and the right to be able to challenge, and that facilitator congruency is crucial to this.

Due to the location of my role within the organisation, I do not have a supervisory role of the students directly within their placement programme area, which may have added another layer of safety for the majority of students. However, for a number of the students I did have a supervisory role as their 'field educator' for their placement, which could raise issues of power, and may have affected their willingness to participate or the incident they chose to explore. I found that those students may have actually enhanced the level of trust they had in me as facilitator, as they knew me. However, power and power relationships need to be acknowledged as an issue and minimised where possible. Healy (2000: 71–73) suggests we cannot distance ourselves from power; rather, we need to be aware of it and its impact.

Results of the formal evaluations

A formal written evaluation was conducted at the end of each set of sessions using a questionnaire incorporating impact, process and outcome questions. A range of themes emerged, which appeared to be intertwined.

Themes

Safe environment

A safe environment was one of the most important aspects of the model identified by students. Thirteen students commented particularly on the value of having a safe environment in which they felt comfortable and supported to undertake their learning about critical reflection, and particularly for presenting their incident. A typical comment was: 'I really enjoyed the process as it was conducted in a comfortable and supportive environment where we were able to learn a process that I think is going to be useful throughout our whole career.'

Role of facilitator

The role of facilitator was seen as very significant, first in generating a safe environment, and second in being skilled in critical reflection and facilitation of the process. This seemed to create another layer of safety for students, which was important given that they were being asked to participate in an unfamiliar process. Third, the role modelling provided by the facilitator meant that students were able to experience the theory in action (Schön, 1987: 255).

Typically students made such comments as: 'The facilitator provided ongoing support, honesty and commitment which built a relationship of trust with all students which was a wonderful role model of professionalism ... it was good knowing that we would not get any negative comments and the atmosphere of being equal.'

Value of group process

Having a group as opposed to individual supervision was also seen as important in assisting students to deconstruct their presented incident. Having a range of inputs and questions provided perspectives of their incident that were different from their own. In this sense, the group broadened and expanded students' perspectives, opening up other possibilities and awareness of assumptions and difference. 'I found the input from other students and the facilitator helpful as they asked questions from angles which I had not thought of ... obtaining other people's perspectives allowed for insight and different ways of looking at an issue and assisted in identifying my underlying assumptions.'

This connected to the opportunity to learn from other people's experiences. Students commented on the learning they gained from hearing other people's incidents and experiences, and the links they could make to their own personal and professional experiences and lives. This seemed to create another dimension of comfort and safety which influenced participants' preparedness to explore and examine their own incident and assumptions. As one said: 'It was important for me to listen to how other people react and see where I also fit my responses to similar issues ... it was really useful to have the chance to be able to listen to other students' presentations and see that some of the issues/anxieties I experienced, others were experiencing the same.'

In this sense, students identified a shared experience and made links between personal experiences and broader global structures. Brookfield (1986: 25) suggests that 'When people hear experiences of other people in a group which are parallel to their own it can create a sense of feeling more comfortable with taking a risk to examine their own assumptions and a sense that personal issues/experiences are linked to shared broader structural issues.'

Given the value seen in the group process, students had mixed views about whether participation should be compulsory. Some valued not being made to feel guilty for not attending, but most thought the sessions were too valuable to miss and that compulsory participation would prevent pressure of other work from becoming the priority.

Importance of the questioning process

Students identified that the questions asked in the critical reflection process were key, achieving a number of outcomes critical to the exploration of their presented incident. The questions asked by group members expanded the perspective they had of their incident by providing new perspectives. Students identified that the questions also assisted them in deconstructing their incident, and examining and unearthing the assumptions that informed their incident and reconstruction of a new theory of practice. Typically, they said: 'The group process involved in this critical reflective technique and the depth and intensity of the questioning enabled me to construct, deconstruct and confront what happened in my presented scenario. I then was able to reconstruct a new perspective of my role within my incident.'

Identification of values and assumptions (making the implicit explicit)

Students particularly commented that the critical reflection process made explicit the implicit assumptions and values they had, which they had not been aware of. Students were often surprised by these and how they shaped their thinking and behaviour: as Yinger (1980: 16) suggests, assumptions become the 'lens and filter for everyday behaviour'. They made links to how these implicit assumptions can impact on their practice and clients and the importance of being aware of this. One commented: 'I learned a lot about myself and my values ... and have identified assumptions that I had not been aware of previously.'

Linking theories to practice

Students commented that the process of critical reflection had enabled them to see how theory and practice linked. They felt the process enabled them to experience critical reflection as a theory in action which made the practice links clearer. They were also able to make practice connections to individual underpinning theories. For example: 'The session on postmodernism taught me the importance of identifying and challenging binary thinking that exists in government and organisational policies, and entrenched negative community perceptions towards welfare dependent families.'

Transferability of skills and awareness to practice

Students identified both the value of transferring their critical reflection skills to practice and that they now felt confident in being able to do this. Some felt this had become part of how they operated in a general way, rather than only in the group. For example: 'These sessions have helped me to identify issues that I have not been aware of previously and they have also provided me with enough understanding of the process to continue to use it throughout my professional and personal life.'

This also connected to thinking about self-care: several students considered that the process of reflecting critically on their experiences encouraged an attitude of self-care and lessened stress. One student commented: 'Assisted me to develop self-care skills and to be able to unpack issues that arise when working with clients or in working life in general.'

Impact on practice and the organisational context

Students highlighted in their evaluations that their participation in critical reflection had provided them with skills to examine their practice, which they considered would improve their work with clients in this or other contexts. Fook (2002: 157) suggests that 'critical reflection is central to the ability to constantly remake practice and practice knowledge and theory in relation to changing contexts. It is a process which allows practitioners to reflect on experience so as to create new knowledge which is transferable to different contexts.' Students considered that workers with these types of skills would be an asset to organisations, particularly those organisations dealing with complex and challenging clients and fields of practice. Miller (2010), in her discussion of the skills and knowledge required by child protection practitioners, emphasises the importance of workers being immersed in professional training, which promotes the skills of critical reflection. A student commented: 'It made me realise how important critical reflection is. With the high demands involved in areas such as child protection work, I think it would be easy to go about our work without stopping to reflect on this. I have learnt to continually ask myself "why am I doing this?" and "what is the purpose?".'

Given the increasing complexity of organisational and client contexts, critical reflection provides practitioners with the ability to stand outside these and examine their practice. One student said: 'I found the critical reflection sessions extremely beneficial in that, when working in the human services field, workers are constantly faced with dilemmas and crises. Learning critical reflection was very relevant in assisting me to deal with this, and to understand and critically reflect on issues from both a worker and client perspective.'

As noted above, students also highlighted in their evaluations that they felt that critical reflection contributed to their self-care. Gibbs (2010) suggests that relationships between workers, organisations and clients are extremely complex and difficult to separate, leading to multiple sources of stress for workers. Therefore it was significant here that students were learning skills that would increase their self-care as professionals.

Fook and Gardner (2007: 149) highlight the question of critical reflection being an organisational rather than an individual process. Reynolds and Vince (2004: 1) examine this in terms of critical reflection focusing on seeking organisational change, with more emphasis on creating collective and organisationally focused processes for critical reflection. Gardner (2007) supports this, proposing that critical reflection can generate change within organisations and is a process that can enable workers to engage with the questions and dilemmas of organisational life. In their evaluations, students highlighted how their experiences reflected the organisational context and how changes in this could alter the culture.

Conclusions and future directions

Conclusions and thoughts for future directions encompass both the model discussed within this chapter for students on placement, and suggestions about how this model could be adapted at an organisational level for staff.

Student placement model

The role of the facilitator appeared to be a critical aspect of the model, with the facilitator being required to have a range of skills. The facilitator must have the ability to maintain a safe environment; be a role model for the theoretical frameworks of critical reflection, using an incident of their own; and support people to take a risk whilst challenging them to examine their assumptions and values in a manner that does not intimidate or judge. The ability of facilitators to ask critical questions, or facilitate these from the group, is crucial to this process. Facilitators must have the ability to simultaneously challenge old modes of thinking whilst providing support and a structure for developing alternative and new ways of thinking and practice (Brookfield, 1984: 74).

Any facilitator of such groups in the future would need to be trained and skilled in critical reflection, with an ability to facilitate and model the process whilst demonstrating a preparedness to be open to take risks and analyse their own assumptions.

Contexts of complexity and change

In the future, in the introductory session I would provide an increased focus on the practice context, which includes not only the client context but also the organisational context. These are the contexts in which the incidents/ dilemmas presented by the students occur and are characterised by increasing uncertainty, change and complexity. Whilst I do focus on this, it would add another level of 'meaning-making' if more time could be dedicated to exploring this with students.

Participation/attendance

I would in the future integrate the critical reflection group into the placement supervision structure, rather than it being seen as an extra activity. This would put a higher expectation on attendance, addressing the issue of work tasks being given priority and disruption to the group process caused by partial attendance. However, this raises issues of power and the disadvantages of involuntary attendance and contributions (Fook and Gardner, 2007: 54–55).

Critical reflection opportunities

I would like to explore the establishment of more critical reflection opportunities and structures within the organisation which are targeted towards staff.

The group model has been highly successful for students and could be adapted for staff. The role of facilitator would be critical to reduce or minimise the impact of power and to establish a safe environment in which to reflect on practice, where staff felt they were not being judged. This model would offer an alternative structure to the current one-on-one supervision, allowing staff to step away from the everyday, taken-for-granted types of processes usually in place within organisations to reflect on practice. This would be particularly useful for challenging contexts such as child protection, where practice is constantly scrutinised.

Being critically reflective would allow a greater depth of exploration of issues and encourage greater self-care as well as more considered practice for clients and possible organisational change. Having staff understand and use critical reflection processes themselves would also enable them to use these more consistently with students to reinforce their learning.

References

Brookfield, S. (1987) *Developing Critical Thinkers: Challenging Adults to Explore Alternative Ways of Thinking and Acting*, San Francisco: Jossey-Bass.

Fook, J. (2008) 'Critical reflection: generating theory from practice', in Pockett, R. and Giles, R. (eds), Sydney: Darlington Press.

Fook, J. and Askeland, G. (2006) 'Challenges of critical reflection: nothing ventured, nothing gained', *Social Work Education*, 1–14.

Fook, J. and Gardner, F. (2007) *Practising Critical Reflection: A Resource Handbook*, Maidenhead: Open University Press.

Gardner, F. (2007) 'Creating a Climate for Change', *International Journal of Knowledge, Culture and Change Management*, 6(7).

Gibbs, J. (2010) 'Window of opportunity', *Victorian Department of Human Services Reflect Newsletter*, 5.

Hawkins, P. and Shohet, R. (2000) *Supervision in the Helping Professions: An Individual, Group and Organizational Approach*, Maidenhead: Open University Press.

Healy, K. (2000) *Social Work Practices: Contemporary Perspectives on Change*, London: Sage.

Mezirow, J. and Associates (2000) *Learning as Transformation: Critical Perspectives on a Theory in Progress*, San Francisco: Jossey-Bass.

Miller, R. (2010) 'The knowledge and skills that child protection practitioners need today', *Advances in Social Work and Welfare Education*, 12 (1)

Reynolds, M.A. and Vince, R. (eds) (2004) *Organizing Reflections*, Aldershot: Ashgate.

Schön, D. (1987) *Educating the Reflective Practitioner*, San Francisco: Jossey-Bass.

Yinger, R.J. (1980) 'Can we really teach them to think?', in Young, R.E. (ed.), *Fostering Critical Thinking*, New Directions for Teaching and Learning 3, San Francisco: Jossey-Bass.

10 Cringe-ical reflection?

Notes on critical reflection and team supervision in a statutory setting

Jeffrey Gordon Baker

When I asked the bright and plucky public sector statutory team I currently manage to dive into the assumption-unsettling reflecting pool of critical reflection, and as they began to reflect upon the incidents that irked and irritated, troubled and preoccupied them in their practice, something happened that I did not expect. Usually an upbeat crew – indeed, remarkably optimistic and enthusiastic for a team of frontline workers, in my experience – the team approached the reflections with characteristically open-minded attitudes and the willingness to learn a new skill. But, despite their generosity of spirit, the sessions always seemed to grow tense and gloomy. And even though they tried to humour me with encouraging feedback, people started making excuses to get out of the sessions, and some members of the team made it quite clear that they would not be at all interested in participating as a reflector in the proverbial 'hot seat'. I had been so excited about introducing critical reflection to the team, but even I was beginning to dread it. It was obvious to everyone that our critical reflections were becoming, well ... *cringe*-ical.

Jan Fook (2002) seems to hint at the potential for this type of phenomenon occurring as part of bringing critical theory to practice, when she quotes Foucault's distinction between that which is *bad* and the less definitive, more evocative concept of that which is *dangerous*. She puts forward that the focus is better placed on the (dangerous) potential of practices (Fook, 2002) – including, I would suggest, critical reflection itself. The notion of *unsettling* that is so crucial to this model of critical reflection is, in fact, a key example of the productive function of this potential. For when assumptions are unsettled, alternative possibilities and perspectives begin to multiply (Fook and Gardner, 2007). However, within a process that has as one of its stated goals the unsettling of assumptions, there is implicit the experience of uncertainty, suspense, of *not* knowing, as well as the inherent possibility that aspects of our professional selves, our practice and its context, will be revealed as problematic or troubling. Feeling exposed as incompetent, like an impostor, suddenly finding oneself in conflict with the cultural values of the agency and experiencing a loss of innocence when we realise that solutions to our dilemmas are not always readily forthcoming: these are among the risks of critical reflection that need to be negotiated (Brookfield, 1995; Fook and Gardner, 2007).

I had set out with the well-intentioned hope of turning the team, with the help of regular reflection, into a shining example of a learning organisation, proving to myself (and the world?) that this could be done, even in the often fraught and embattled environment of statutory work. Indeed, this practice setting seemed the perfect place in which to introduce critical reflection as a tool for re-finding our ethical selves within a personal/professional value base and for renewing our theories of practice accordingly, even as we traversed the bureaucratic terrain of work within the state system. But in my enthusiasm, I discovered that care needs to be taken as, paradoxically, the experience of approaching the productively 'dangerous' risks of reflection can also have unforeseen destabilising effects that not only unsettle, but threaten to derail the whole project.

So this is my personal reflection, in which I use the experience of navigating this landscape as an incident by way of which to reflect upon my own assumptions about the statutory work environment and the way in which I have introduced critical reflection as a group supervision tool within it.

***

Prior to joining this team, I had the experience of facilitating critical reflection only within educational contexts, running groups as part of a newly qualified social worker programme and as part of the reflective practice module of a Master's programme in professional studies, and although participants in each of these groups brought incidents for reflection that dealt directly with their experience in practice, neither group took place in the practice context itself. Furthermore, I was interested in using the process specifically for team supervision, as a way to identify the professional issues that were important to the individual workers and to the team as a whole (Fook and Gardner, 2007). In this way, I hoped that the reflection groups would be a means by which I could get to know the team of workers I would be managing. I was also motivated by what I saw as the opportunity to bring reflection into the high-intensity, high-stress world of statutory child protection, a practice environment often viewed as more reactive than reflective.

By way of background, I should explain that my taking up this managerial role is a recent and somewhat unexpected development in my personal career trajectory. Although I have a background in statutory child care work, I had been purposefully moving away from frontline practice, in the direction of social work education, practice-assessing student social workers on their work placements and leading workshops. In addition to this self-employed work, I was in a part-time role as training and learning development coordinator for a pilot programme in the children's services department of a local government department. I was just beginning to piece together a new shape to my career when news came of drastic cuts to public sector funding

(Wintour and Mulholland, 2010). Following word of these forthcoming austerity measures, the educational programmes that I was developing, which were previously seen as the bold way forward, were given decidedly less priority. Times were changing and, although I knew that I still wanted to pursue a more academic career, the climate felt too unstable to continue in part-time freelance work, especially as I was just starting out in this new direction. I felt that I needed to shore up my personal resources by doing some agency work back on the frontline. In short, the plan was to save up money while I explored the possibility of PhD study.

I shortly found myself placed by my employment agency in a management position on a referral and assessment child protection team, and shortly after that was offered the permanent position of team manager. Ironically, this was exactly the type of thing I had been steering my career away from. And yet fortuitously I found that my new team members – despite the fact that they are incredibly busy and at times overworked, in an area of the city with high profile and serious cases in its recent history – were remarkably enthusiastic, energetic and motivated to improve their practice. It was largely for this reason that I decided to take the permanent position despite my previous intention to remain on short-term contract.

There were practical adjustments to be made to the critical reflection model from the outset, departing slightly from the process outlined by Fook and Gardner (2007). As mentioned, the area of the city and the department's function make for an extremely busy workplace, and despite their goodwill and positive attitude about learning and development, figuring out how to introduce a regular time-consuming activity into the already hectic schedule of the team was to prove complicated. But where there's a will there's a way, and my first move was to schedule a team away-day at which to deliver the introductory session on the theory behind the model and the process. During this session, I modelled the process by presenting an incident of my own for reflection.

In undertaking my model reflection, it became clear that, even if they felt they were treading on new ground and feeling uncertain about whether they were doing it right, the team did understand the basics as set out in the introductory session. Many of the same issues that I had seen arise with other groups came up as the group negotiated the learning curve, becoming increasingly familiar with the process. The necessary role of the facilitator is evident, as the group initially needs to be redirected from innocently making judgements and getting caught up with the situation as they imagine they might personally have experienced it, rather than the story as constructed by the person reflecting. I find that this often takes place when group members identify and empathise with the person reflecting, and is part of a supportive or even protective impulse being activated within the group. This necessitates the need for reminders about support and affirmation needing to be limited and utilised by way of encouraging the reflecting participant to come to their own conclusions and to focus on those aspects of their story that are relevant to them, rather than mirroring the reflector's story with identifications from group members' own practice.

The introduction at the away-day went much like the other groups I had led, although the team later gave feedback that the 'lecture' portion had reminded them of lectures at university, and wasn't as enjoyable as the reflection session itself, to which they responded more favourably. This was an early indication of the difference between facilitating critical reflection in the workplace as part of the ongoing life of the team, as opposed to working with a group gathered explicitly for the purpose of education or training. The latter type of group has, in my experience, tended to express appreciation for the introductory lecture as being what they feel they 'are there for', and may approach the actual reflection with a bit more trepidation, it being an experiential activity outside the realm of didactic learning. This highlights the way in which critical reflection tends to – depending upon how you look at it – either bridge the gap between practice and theory/education, or fall into it, since it doesn't squarely fit in either camp. This is possibly the reason why the function and process of reflection generally is, at times, contested and portrayed as being vague and unconvincingly defined (Ixer, 2011).

In choosing my own incident for reflection, I purposely selected something that had come up in the context of my practice when I had been a frontline worker and that explicitly pointed to the rigidity of the statutory setting, in which a focus on procedure often consumes any consideration of the quality of experience of clients, or workers for that matter. During the away-day I stated that it was my express goal to reconnect the work we do to the values of the profession as a whole. I have often employed the metaphor of a factory, insisting that even though we do relatively short-term work on the referral and assessment team, and are often under pressure to move cases along quickly, I do not want to succumb to the feeling that we, or the children and families with whom we are engaged, are like workers and products along a swiftly moving assembly line of case disposition.

Interestingly, in an article presenting qualitative research about the experience of frontline state social workers in the first decade of the New Labour government in the UK, Chris Jones (2001: 553) discovers to his surprise that for 'the first time in my experience I was listening to social workers describe their work as if they were in a factory'. His research shows workers' disillusion increasing as a function of business management models being implemented to measure productivity in social care work. Ten years on from the publication of this article, many of the same instruments drive statutory work, and I was (and still am) keen that my team should not lose sight of the individual experiences of either our clients or ourselves as professionals, with a value base underpinning the profession we have chosen. Now, the scaling back of public sector resources and the management strategies that came with New Labour (Jones, 2001) have been combined with 'permanent' cuts to resources with which the Conservative government has informed the public services they will have to live with in the long term (Wintour and

Mulholland, 2010), leaving frontline workers like my team with even fewer options for supporting their clients, but with the same pressure to constantly 'manage' risk. It is possible with hindsight to see how the process might turn on itself in an atmosphere that is already hostile to the experience of individuals, both staff and clients, supporting the swift output of the system itself over human relationships (Jones, 2001). Somewhat aware of this from the first, I was clear with my own manager that my taking up this permanent managerial role was contingent on my ability to use reflection as a tool to highlight the contradictions and ethical dilemmas that are part and parcel of this milieu.

Following the away-day in which the model was introduced, it was some weeks before we had the opportunity to sit down with another member of the team to undertake our first official reflection session. This practical concern was to prove an ongoing challenge: how to ensure on a busy team, part of whose function is to deal with emergencies and a high turnover of cases, that reflection sessions take place closely enough together for the group to maintain focus and a connection to the process and its relevance to day-to-day practice. It was important to me that critical reflection be a staple activity of the team, a regularly occurring team development project. For this reason I decided that we would do stages one and two within the same roughly hour-and-a-half-long session with a short break in between, and I scheduled team meetings twice a month in which the sessions would take place. I spoke to individual members of the team, in our one-to-one supervision sessions, about the possibility of taking part as a reflecting participant, and assisted them in identifying incidents they might use as raw material for reflection.

In the first session I gave out handouts with the stage one and two questions printed on them as a way to remind the group of the process they had learned at the away-day. There was a tentative feeling at the beginning of the session, and I felt unusually nervous myself, more so than I remember feeling even at the first session I ever facilitated, or with any of the groups I have previously worked with. I admit that this feeling on my part took me by surprise. I did not have a chance to think about it at the time, but upon subsequent reflection, I think that it was at least partially to do with the personal investment I was making in the sessions – making the use of critical reflection, and the impact I hoped it would have on my participation in a work environment (frontline/ statutory) that I had effectively 'sworn off', so to speak, a condition of my allowing myself to accept the position of team manager. It now seems obvious that I was probably feeling nervous because I had made the stakes for myself very high indeed.

Questions that have the effect of being judgemental, due to their reliance on either speculation about the reflector's experience of the incident or the personal experience of the questioner, are not unusual with a group that is not yet used to the process, but in this situation – which was new for me as well – I found it difficult to reframe them without seeming to shut down the team member altogether, causing them to withdraw into a kind of quiet shame. I found it very difficult to tolerate the long silences between questions, and each redirection that I made to questions from the group seemed to require a long explanation with examples and counter-examples to back it up. The team member participating as the reflector was answering thoughtfully and with openness and honesty, but the group itself seemed stymied at points, and I felt the pressure of time constraint and the frequent awkward silences raising the temperature in the room. Progress was slow – or at least this was my perception in the heat of the moment – and at one point I resorted to instructing them to just read out questions directly from the sheet of paper I had handed them. Of course, this felt awkward and forced, and the whole session ran very long, the better part of two hours. But given the generosity of the reflector, it did amount to a rich experience with regard to content. The individual was able to isolate what he felt were the main assumptions and reformulate a theory of practice in light of these.

But when we took time to debrief afterwards, the group members seemed nervous and were halting in their responses to my questions about how they had experienced the session. They seemed to find it hard to articulate – as did I – the nature of what had felt uncomfortable about the process. One member of the team ventured something along the lines of 'I'm not sure I liked it'. And someone else mentioned that the questions seemed tricky, as if they were designed to fool the person reflecting into revealing something – which, ironically, in a way they are, just without the implied dark edge of deceit spoiling the atmosphere.

I'm usually fairly confident in my various roles as a team leader/supervisor and teacher/practice educator, but in this situation, in which they were suddenly combined, I felt like a sham. I must have looked very disappointed because during the debrief, and in individual supervision sessions with several workers in the following weeks, a number of people tried their best to speak positively about the session and the idea of reflection in general, qualifying this by saying that they didn't feel they were doing it correctly and were unclear about what the questions were trying to achieve. It was a testament to their kindness that most of them were so polite about it, but I knew that the responsibility lay with me, and my inability to structure the work of reflection in such a way that the team felt secure within it. In short, the questions had worked and the session was productive in unsettling assumptions, but the problem was that we all remained ... unsettled. And I didn't know what to do about it.

I think it is significant that all the reflector-participants brought critical incidents related either directly or indirectly to elements of the statutory workplace that constrain and affect the way we work with clients. One worker addressed his feeling that the prescribed interventions that we had to carry out with the police were rarely tailored to the needs of the family, but were driven by procedure, often feeling as if they were doing more harm than good, despite the fact that they are ostensibly in place to protect children. Another worker's incident related to a complaint that had been made against her by the mother of a young person remanded by the court into local authority care. Her reflection revealed her assumptions about her power-lessness over this mother's negative experience, since the actions being complained about had been in the context of procedures outside her (the worker's) control. Another felt that she was forced into being more harsh and punitive than she would have liked in expressing her concerns about a situation in a large, multi-agency meeting, due to the formality of proceedings seeming to dictate that family and worker 'take sides' in opposition to one another. All the participants' reflections contained elements that were both emotional and professionally personal; most touched upon personal theories about their reasons for undertaking this kind of work and the aspects of the job that got in the way of these. Significantly, none of the participants revealed information about their private lives outside the workplace, and on several occasions they were able to draw boundaries with regard to certain avenues of questioning with which they did not feel completely comfortable.

Following the first reflection session, people had repeatedly mentioned their fearfulness about asking the wrong question, or not knowing what kinds of question to ask. For this reason, and because the first reflection had run over time, I continued to institute the practice of having the group ask questions directly from the printed handout, making it even more formal by having them go around the circle, each of them asking a question in turn. Even as I write this, I realise how ridiculous it was to micro-manage the sessions in this way. But my assumption was that it was the only way to both deal with the problem of limited time and avoid the experience of participants feeling embarrassed at not knowing exactly what to ask.

My assumption, upon reflection, was that I was desperate for the sessions to yield results, so I effectively distilled the model down to the questions and answers, creating a streamlined process designed to get results in the quickest way possible. The feedback reflected this, with members of the team reporting that they felt the formal elements I had introduced (reading off the paper, asking questions in turn) had eclipsed the natural flow of the group and contrasted with the normally casual and conversational spirit of the team, making the mood stilted. Amazingly, I realise that what I have done is to replicate, in the process of reflection itself, the very aspects of statutory work that I was hoping to counteract by introducing reflection into the team. Time-scales and 'tick-box' social work that have been imposed on the practice of state social work were meant to somehow quantify and quality-control a practice that is meant to be about caring relationships between professionals and those they serve (Jones, 2001). In 'streamlining' the process of reflection in order to save time and maximise results, I was recreating this same overwrought and inhuman atmosphere within the reflective space.

This replication of the pressurised conditions I was hoping to alleviate through the use of reflection is one way of understanding the phenomenon of what I have referred to as *cringe*-ical reflection, which overcast our team supervision. But another aspect that must not be avoided is my own participa-tion in power as I led the team into the use of critical reflection. In gathering feedback on the sessions, several people offered bravely that the discomfort felt might have something to do with – not *me* personally, they hastened to qualify! – but with my being their manager and supervisor as well as the facilitator of the reflection sessions. I assume this comment to be important for two reasons. Firstly, it highlights my role as being potentially representative of the strict and unyielding state social work system, and therefore the need to approach my facilitation of the reflections with this potential pitfall in mind. But, para-doxically, for me on a personal level it reinforces how the whole experience had made me feel like an impostor, like someone whose own ambivalence about the strictures of the work setting, coupled with the seeming inability to help his team negotiate their way through them, effectively disqualifies me from my own professional role.

Brookfield (1995) speaks about this 'impostor syndrome' as one of the risks of critical reflection, and suggests the importance of naming it in order to diminish its paralysing power. He also refers to the risk of what he terms 'cultural suicide', in which the practice and even the overt enthusiasm for the transformative process of critical reflection can alienate co-workers and lead to the marginalisation of its proponents, who can be viewed as acting subversively, irritatingly raising difficult and uncomfortable questions rather than being seen as agents of positive change. These risks were clearly intersecting factors in the dynamic of my situation in my team. One possible scenario that these risks suggest is that I came on too strong, using my team-leader position to decide unilaterally to implement the groups, which I then subsequently micro-managed – my own enthusiasm for the method, coupled with my power to enforce it in the way I thought best, producing a feeling of overwhelm for the group. Another perspective is that it was the productive use of the method itself that laid bare certain theories of practice about our work that may have hit too close to home too quickly, and I was too busy being excited about the use of critical reflection to notice these feelings and help us all to debrief about them.

But the truth – somewhere in the middle as usual – was that I did notice. Indeed, the tense and anxious reaction of the team inside the sessions and their avoidance later made me feel that I had failed them. Once confident that I was bringing a new era of reflective practice to my small corner of the state social work world, I suddenly felt that I had no idea what I was talking about and, in turn, it made me feel that I had been 'beaten' by the bureaucratic machine I had so hopefully deployed critical reflection to combat.

I think I did the right thing when I publicly named my feelings about the groups, acknowledging openly with the team my recognition that the experience had been more intense – in a negative way – than I had expected, and asking their opinion as to what they thought might help. The work has now become more diversely focused: we have developed 'team goals' to guide all of our work, including those aspects related to supporting each other and developing our skills, and critical reflection sessions – in a more relaxed format – figure into this plan. We have dispensed with reading out the questions off the printed page, and the first and second stages of the process tend to blend into one another more seamlessly in reflection sessions that are no more than an hour in length.

I have asked the reflector and the group to focus primarily on four main areas: the incident, asking the individual reflecting to isolate as closely as possible what they feel was the most critical part of the situation for them; assumptions of the individual about the incident and where these might come from; alternative perspectives on these assumptions; and how all of the above relate to the individual's experience of power in the incident and, following on from this, their assumptions about their participation in power generally. I have found that gently steering the discussion in these directions has been enough to keep us on track and focused within a tighter timeframe. And the group – including new members who were not present for the introductory session or any of our later discussions – have become increasingly comfortable with formulating their own questions in order to draw out material around these areas of focus. We are also starting to rotate the facilitator role, which will give me a chance occasionally to do a reflection myself, outside the context of demonstrating the model or facilitating. This will hopefully reinforce reflection as an activity that we are doing together, rather than something I am teaching them.

Indeed, one of the main assumptions that I have unearthed through reflecting on the experience of using critical reflection with the team relates to the way in which the *managerial* role influences and interacts with the *social work* role in the statutory practice setting. Despite best efforts to at least nominally recognise social work values and ethics across the board in frontline teams, and paying lip service to 'anti-oppressive practice', state social work is still characterised by a sharp divide between practitioners and managers. And this 'them-and-us' culture can lead to the 'proletarianisation' of the workers, meaning that state social work can have the effect of turning social workers into a subjugated class of labourers doing production-line work rather than forming working relationships (Jones, 2001: 559). The deleterious effect of this power imbalance is what I would call an *institutional* assumption, institutional in the sense that it appeared and influenced the supervisory relationship as it is structured and viewed specifically in the statutory environment. I feel this is evidenced at least in part by the very different reception I had when facilitating reflections in educational settings as an educator, as opposed to when I was the leader of a team in a managerial role.

The use of critical reflection in our team is still a work in progress, but the reflection I have done in the process of writing this chapter has helped me to make explicit some of its risks as they pertain to my role as the manager of a statutory team, and my participation in this position of power. Implicit within this are assumptions about the way power functions in the state social work system. For example, it was remarkable to discover, through reflection, the way in which some of my actions as the manager–facilitator of our sessions effectively recreated the dehumanising function of the statutory system, and how the team's reactions to this were similar to the reactions of frontline workers to bureaucratic and managerial structures being imposed on social work in the public sector. It is beyond the scope of the present discussion whether critical reflection within the frontline statutory setting can bring about *emancipatory change*, assisting workers to overcome their feelings of disempowerment (Morley, 2011) brought on by work in this system – especially in the current stringent and 'streamlined' climate. But addressing head-on the risks that can attend the use of critical reflection in the state social work environment seems a vital and necessary step in the direction of its *emancipatory possibilities* (Fook, 2004), for both individual workers and the wider culture of the social work profession.

References

Brookfield, S.D. (1995) *Becoming a Critically Reflective Teacher*, San Francisco: Jossey-Bass.

Fook, J. (2002) *Social Work: Critical Theory and Practice*, London: Sage.

——(2004) 'Critical reflection and transformative possibilities', in Davies, L. and Leonard, P. (eds), *Social Work in a Corporate Era: Practices of Power and Resistance*, Aldershot: Ashgate, 16–30.

Fook, J. and Gardner, F. (2007) *Practising Critical Reflection: A Resource Handbook*, Maidenhead: Open University Press.

Ixer, G. (2011) '"There's no such thing as reflection" ten years on', *Journal of Practice Teaching and Learning*, 10(1): 75–93.

Jones, C. (2001) 'Voices from the front line: state social workers and New Labour', *British Journal of Social Work*, 31: 547–62.

Morley, C. (2011) 'How does critical reflection develop possibilities for emancipatory change? An example from an empirical research project', *British Journal of Social Work*, 41: 1–20.

Wintour, P. and Mulholland, H. (2010) 'David Cameron warns public sector cuts will be permanent', *The Guardian* [online], 3 August, www.guardian.co.uk/politics/2010/aug/03/david-cameron-public-sector-cuts-permanent?INTCMP=SRCH

11 Learning to play hide-and-seek with pink elephants

Belinda Hearne

Introduction

Adult learning is sometimes more complex and uncomfortable than the learning experiences of childhood. Critical reflection as a learning mode has provided me with a tool that can find a way through unhelpful constraints regarding personal practices and assumed theories about life, work and people; it sustains my work as a manager and provides encouragement.

In this chapter I will show how it has assisted my learning and influenced my continued integration of management practices, theory and values. My journey began through a Master's research thesis (Hearne, 2007) which utilised critical reflection as described by Fook and Gardner (2007). Their framework assisted me to identify my own hidden assumptions that were influencing my theory of management and, in turn, affected my management practices.

The deconstruction of critical incidents revealed themes in terms of my theoretical construction of power and its operations which limited my options for practice, particularly where anxiety was underlying conflict. In reconstructing my ideas, I opened up new possibilities for practice and a way to use critical reflection with my colleagues. In essence, this has led to a process of emancipation, a freeing up of me in my role, and an increased understanding of the experience of change and my own and my colleagues' experience of anxiety at work. This, in turn, has led to an understanding of the constraining force that anxiety has on learning when managing complex organisational environments.

Organisational background

The particular organisational example I am going to use is a community health setting in a rural community. In small Australian rural towns such as this one, community health is a complex workplace. Small teams with limited resources and management infrastructure are accountable to multiple government departments. The rural environment presents unique challenges, with little public transport connecting towns, high unemployment, isolation and few partner agencies. Each community health program team is driven by

conflicting government department philosophies for the delivery of diverse services across mental health, family services, drug and alcohol, health promotion,
allied health, and a range of other varied program areas. Programs are
expected to deliver across the life span, meeting particular needs of people across
multiple continuums of health and illness, within frameworks of direct service,
case work, community development, health promotion and administration.

The pace of change driven by globalisation brings a requirement for organisations to adjust rapidly and flexibly, and to be innovative; the complex
demands it places on community health is shared by many in the modern
workplace. In recent decades this has resulted in increased complexity, rapid
program change driven at system level by changed organisational theoretical
discourses, and new environmental market forces. These, in turn, impact on
organisations demanding greater flexibility in their efforts to adapt to change
and to learn, both individually and collectively (Senge, 1990; Gould, 2000;
Gould and Baldwin, 2004; Cressey et al., 2006; Gardner, 2006).

Rapid change and the destabilising nature of modern work bring unpredictability, role fluidity and greater accountability, and require flexibility
(Cressey et al., 2006). Practitioners with whom I work often express their
sense of 'loss of control' over their work, and anxiety in relation to change.
These experiences have emotional effects that affect organisations' ability to
change. The effect is one in which complex multifactorial issues have an
impact on organisations' ability to 'organise' (Vince, 2001).

Learning about the power of pink elephants

As a manager of counselling and health teams, and from the process of my
own critical reflection journey, I wanted to understand organisational dynamics
and their crucial role in either constraining or facilitating organisations' efforts
to adapt and change. My attention had been focused upon the influence of
power and emotions at work, and how the related dynamics affect organising
in organisations. I was curious about my participation in these dynamics,
and ways to promote rather than detract from learning that occurs organisationally. In my own critical reflection process of investigation into management
power and its operations, I read Vince (2001), whose ideas I found helpful.
His writing challenges managers to reflect on their use of power and risk,
making visible emotion in the workplace. Vince states that:

> Organisational dynamics are constructed from the interaction between
> emotions (such as envy, guilt, anxiety and emotions that are avoided or
> ignored), and power that create the social and political context within
> which both learning and organising can take place.
>
> (Vince, 2001: 1326)

At work, emotions such as anxiety, frustration or envy are not comfortable
and invite avoidance. The metaphor of the 'pink elephant in the room' is

commonly used to describe a problem which organisational members may ignore or avoid. The ways in which dynamics, influenced by power and emotion, affect communication between organisational members will influence the organisation's ability to adapt and change. Using critical reflection to attend to the collective experience of working together and observing the way organisational communication occurs can provide insight into how and what the organisation learns.

Vince asserts that the emotional aspect within organisations is often difficult for organisational members to negotiate. The focus of my research was on anxiety as an emotion and its impact on learning in organisations. Anxiety can be triggered at both the individual and organisational level. Individuals may experience anxiety due to 'having to say something difficult or challenging, by the effects of unwanted decisions, by the pressures of an unfamiliar task' (Vince, 2002: 78). For organisational groups, anxiety may be triggered by 'external deadlines, demands, shifts of decision making that occur in other parts of the organisation, or through interaction across inter-group boundaries' (ibid). In each of these scenarios, the 'individual or group is faced with a strategic moment, where anxiety can either be held and worked through towards some form of insight, or it can ignored and avoided, creating a "willing ignorance"' (Vince, 2002: 79).

Promoting or restraining learning

Vince describes two communication pathways that may occur at the strategic moment when anxiety is triggered. Both communication pathways occur in dynamic and strategic ways at the individual and subgroup levels, and represent the ways in which learning is promoted or restrained, with change effected as an outcome.

In communication that promotes learning, the strategic moment in which anxiety occurs creates uncertainty. The uncertainty, if held long enough, allows for risks to be taken. 'Risk and the struggle that makes possible, provides a potential for new knowledge or insight' (Vince, 2002: 79). In communication that restrains learning, 'uncertainty cannot be held and anxiety promotes denial or avoidance of emotions that seem too difficult to address'; such communication is characterised by defensive resistance and, ultimately, 'willing ignorance' (ibid).

Managers, anxiety and critical reflection

This section explores my use of critical reflection in a workplace research project that assisted us to inquire into, and develop understandings about, the relationship between anxiety and organisational learning. The chosen chapter title emerged from the research group who named themselves the 'pink elephant club', and aims to make light of the interplay between both avoiding (hide) and desiring (seek) learning in the way we relate at work.

By the time the research project emerged, my critical reflection journey had already helped me to reconstruct ideas and develop a theory of practice about the operations of power in organisations, which I described for myself as a 'cautionary use of power'. Alongside this, organisational processes had been introduced utilising critical reflection for counselling supervision groups. In these groups, taking risks in communication was already occurring in relation to utilising the Fook and Gardner (2007) model.

The framework from Vince helped me practice a cautionary use of power at work by offering understandings about how and when I chose to contribute to either promoting or restraining learning.

Formulation of the research project and design

The exploration of anxiety was built on my own individual critical reflection learning. Critical reflection supervision groups existed for two years prior to this project, and helped provide a safe context for those staff who volunteered to make an enquiry, together with myself as manager, about the role of organisational anxiety. The project question emerged in conversation with staff members after I noticed that a significant workplace confidential conflict was being discussed informally. This was the entry point for conversations about conflict at work. Some organisational members, who had become familiar with the use of critical reflection for their clinical work, had a shared framework with me in being curious about aspects of organisational life. Initially, I asked whether they would join me in examining the nature of conflict at work. This was not something they decided they could do; conflict was definitely too risky to discuss. However, our consultative conversations resulted in agreement that we would examine the topic of anxiety.

While practising a 'cautionary use of power', the particular question that I wanted to explore with my colleagues was: How does action research design and critical reflection method, as a process for collective learning about anxiety, influence, over time, the theories surrounding anxiety that organisational members may hold?

The Fook and Gardner model was adapted for this project. Counselling and community development supervision groups were already providing a structure through which individual organisational members identified their own critical incident and worked through these in confidential supervision groups. The research project introduced organisational members who had not been exposed to critical reflection supervision groups at a broader organisational level. It also provided an opportunity to work collectively on the theme of anxiety, utilising individual critical incidents to make visible a common experience across the different teams.

The research design utilised a qualitative action research model linking enquiry with learning and change. The action research model parallels the processes identified in learning organisation literature for assisting organisational members to use reflective practice. This reflective practice process is described as a learning cycle of reflecting, thinking, feeling, connecting, deciding and doing (Senge, 1990). The critical elements of reflection that were of interest were the collective exploration and questioning of assumptions and the revealing of power relations with the intention of action to change in the interests of emancipation (Reynolds and Vince, 2004). The methodology I chose provided an opportunity to utilise a critically reflective method (Fook and Gardner, 2007), linked to an action research process as a means of developing a collective experience that could be described as organisational learning. My aim was to assist us understand the theories we held about anxiety by reflecting on the experiences of anxiety, and to discover whether critical reflection would influence our behaviour in relation to anxiety and support emotional and behavioural emancipation.

The organisation's senior management team and an external ethics committee approved the research proposal, and I advertised for and recruited voluntary participants through open invitations emailed to all staff. Twelve potential participants, from a variety of programs, responded and attended an introductory meeting.

At the first meeting I led a discussion about anxiety, its relationship to organisational learning, and its usefulness as representative of an emotion that might be used to trial a collective critical reflection process. I provided information concerning the structure of the groups and participant rights to privacy and confidentiality. Nine employees, out of the twelve who volunteered, were selected on the basis of providing a diverse representation across the organisation's program areas.

Data was collected using focus groups of two hours' duration. Groups were semi-structured, drawing on the practices of critical reflection (Fook, 2002a, b; Fook and Gardner, 2007) to provide a framework for interviews and gathering data. The introductory hour for explanation and four focus group sessions spanned a five-month period with a commitment of nine hours for participants. Data was collected via audiotapes and scribed information.

Critical reflection practice provided a framework to assist participants to describe understandings and identify individual assumptions about anxiety, which helped describe the collective meaning and effect of anxiety in the organisation. In the first session, participants identified scenarios where they experienced anxiety and collectively brainstormed the effects of anxiety on their thoughts and behaviour. Each participant chose a metaphor that best described anxiety for them.

In between sessions, participants were asked to notice situations where they experienced anxiety, and their response. Participants were provided with transcripts after each session to assist their reflections, verify meanings and document accumulating data. I was interested in whether the data was capturing understandings from sequential groups. Were there further understandings that needed to be added? Was anything of importance omitted? Was this what participants assumed would emerge? How did this inform us in relation to anxiety and organisational learning?

Before the final session, I examined the data in relation to the literature, and selected Vince's framework described earlier. This was provided to participants, who evaluated it against their experiences and generated meanings.

In the final session, we collected further data regarding participants' reflections on anxiety. We evaluated the usefulness of the critical reflection process in terms of: changes in thinking; recommendations for further use; or reluctance to use the process organisationally. Recommendations for change were acknowledged and a process was developed for how the findings would be disseminated.

Data analysis

I transcribed audiotaped data collected from focus groups. I utilised a thematic analysis to construct coded information that formed the basis of categories of analysis according to themes relating to anxiety (Boyatzis, 1998). Coded categories constructed in the first session were refined and expanded over following sessions and provided to participants for further reflection, development of themes, and recommendations for change. 'Theory building from practice' was utilised in this research, and in the first three sessions we gained an understanding of a collective 'theory in use' (Argyris and Schön, 1996) by drawing from the individual shared experiences of participants. In the fourth session, the knowledge generated from the experiences described by participants was evaluated by them against Vince's ideas on the relationship anxiety has to either restraining or promoting learning.

What did we learn about anxiety?

The theory of anxiety that participants held changed over time. A definition of critical reflection is useful to revisit in discussing how it supported the changes.

> Reflective practice encourages workers to stop and think about their practice ... taking into account what they think and feel about it. The process includes analysing practice in the sense of exploring assumptions and values that influence how they work so that workers look at these consciously and consider the implications of this for practice. The critical element adds an expectation of exploring practice in the context of the social system that it operates.
>
> (Gardner, 2006: 19)

Participants experienced changes over the life of the project in their theory and practice in relation to anxiety. The third and fourth sessions provided the strongest evidence in relation to answering the research question: that is, how the process of action research design and critical reflection method influences collective learning about anxiety over time and changes theories surrounding anxiety that organisational members may hold.

Analysing data transcripts allowed us collectively to critically reflect on previous sessions and the assumptions and values that underpinned our responses. Each session deconstructed anxiety and built on thinking that emerged from the previous one. For example, in the first session, participants generated metaphors such as 'the pink elephant in the room' to describe their experience of anxiety. In the second session, when examining the transcripts, participants questioned 'How could someone not notice a pink elephant?'.

The research provided a safe environment where participants first noticed how they responded to anxiety; and second questioned their underlying assumptions and values. For example, the negative construction of other colleagues became visible. The following example indicates the early stages of change of theory in use, where participants reflected upon the way judgements or criticism of colleagues could be understood using alternative explanations such as anxiety.

> I am just thinking about the hassles and anxieties I have with child protection workers, and you talking about that leaves me thinking about the workers, where some of what I have tagged as incompetence is actually their anxiety around what is going on as well ... I have never thought about them being anxious.

By the third session, anxiety caused by conflict emerged. Participants agreed that although conflict was anxiety-provoking, this was also a normal part of organisational life.

> I think we all bring a whole lot of fears and fragilities and anxiety around conflict. At one level we don't want conflict to occur, but at another we see it as inevitable and something we have to deal with and manage.

Participants began noticing that emotions were not made visible in organisational meetings. One participant was considering taking risks to find the 'courage' to name how they were feeling. Another was reflecting on the importance of naming emotions instead of blaming others. These examples demonstrate a shift in the group from theorising to changing practices.

> I remember our very first session here. We were saying that anxiety was this pink elephant or whatever. It is around, and we all hold it – it's expressed to some degree but we never name it – we could be naming instead of blaming others.

Different views were held regarding conflict. One participant doubted that having conflict with a manager would bring about change. This shifted the focus to the hierarchical nature of power relations. In Vince's view, these conversations are important to the reflective process because they bring to light ways in which power operates to restrain or promote learning. Safety to have conflict and the power to influence change were important themes influencing whether or not participants were willing to enter into conflict.

> What makes it unsafe for me is the stress it causes myself individually, and that stress characterises my workplace. The cost is my stress, and the benefit, well, there isn't any because there is no change … if there was more opportunity to change then you would be prepared to have more conflict.

A recurring theme was the lack of clarity of the strategic plan's vision and organisational goals. Participants debated the complexity of developing a shared vision, organisational goals and the nature of the competing discipline-based discourses that made this process difficult. Participants identified that there were no structures through which discussion of competing discourses could occur that could assist the organisation to reflect on these differences. Here we see change as organisational levels of analysis emerge.

Prior to the final session, I reviewed the literature to find a framework against which to understand emerging data and support participants to synthesise their ideas. Vince's representation of learning as promoted or restrained was provided in order to elicit participants' views on whether this fitted with their experiences. In discussion of the model, participants were able to identify when and how, in the presence of anxiety, they moved between promoted or restrained learning.

Vince's framework assisted participants to identify the existing organisational structures where learning was promoted. One area was the critical reflection supervision groups that were embedded in the organisation twelve months previously. Four of the participants had been involved in these groups.

> That (promoting learning) reminds me of the stuff we do in critical reflection supervision. We go in with some uncertainty, we take a huge risk in talking about a critical incident – I wouldn't talk about it anywhere else – then we all struggle with it – not just the person who brings it in.

Participants could identify how the supervision structures might be useful in promoting learning:

> as an individual, you are more likely to be positioned in the restrained learning, but if there are structures and group processes in place, you are more likely to be in the promoting learning. You can start working as teams rather than individuals.

Participants identified limitations to the supervision groups and began to look for other structures that might provide alternatives.

The critical reflection supervision model does provide that space and allows us to look at our anxiety, but it is anxiety around practice rather than around organisational issues ... we are in the midst of accreditation and we have these working teams looking at standards. I am looking for opportunities within the organisational structure and that is one of them.

Restrained learning was recognised as a place of safety in which to avoid conflict, but also a process that could create inflexibility.

When individuals play in that (restrained learning), or management play in that, nothing changes. Management hold onto their position, the organisation holds on to its position, the individual holds on to their position. There is no change, no movement and there is no learning.

In the final group, a serious conflict situation in the organisation emerged as a point of discussion. The critical reflection practice used in previous sessions provided a foundation for development of safety: the use of participant skills and shared practice knowledge enabled participants to challenge each other and to articulate assumptions. Two participant subgroups emerged: those who had direct knowledge and experience of the conflict from within a program area, and those who had known nothing about the conflict until the final stages, when certain aspects became public in the organisation. This second subsystem was affected by the outcome of the conflict and concerned about agency procedures. Although there was no overt hostility, emotions were expressed and processed. Essentially, the two subsystems engaged in conflict and worked through this together. The communication was representative of a promoting learning process. One participant used Vince's framework to start the conversation by saying:

I am going to name the pink elephant because in the last few months there was a lot of anxiety around an agency conflict and I behaved in this [restrained learning] because I couldn't deal with it. I denied that it was in the room. I denied it and avoided it.

Both positions were discussed from each subsystem's perspective. Participants used Vince's framework to support the conversation with comments indicating at what point they retreated into restrained learning and why. Feelings of exclusion, confusion and fear that different subgroups experienced at different points in the process were expressed. Meetings with management and different perspectives on the impact of these meetings for different groups were shared. Assumptions were challenged and new understandings emerged. The problems associated with talking about the issue when staff integrity and rights to privacy were involved, and the experience of talking about the issues as 'gossip', highlighted for participants the tensions inherent in the nature of organisational confidentiality.

During this process, I documented the experience from the perspective of the participants. However, my own learning was also significant. The most powerful element for me was the ability of the process described above to create enough safety for organisational members to discuss a conflict situation that we all knew that I, as manager, had intimate experience and knowledge of, whilst also maintaining confidentiality. I learned about the influence of rights such as confidentiality both to protect individual organisational members, but also to create the ingredients for conspiracy theories based on assumptions that emerged to fill in gaps in understanding. I realised that the participants had formed subgroups holding the 'for-and-against' dichotomised points of view. As they discussed what they knew, I became the audience (with my own process), watching the ripple effects played out beyond my immediate involvement.

The research made visible how complex organisations are, and how we create structures that support aspects of organisational life to remain invisible by avoiding or ignoring them. Less visible aspects can flourish, creating difficulties between subgroups. This process also challenged the 'them-and-us' idea of manager and worker. This experience has invited my ongoing observation of how this emerges, the different roles we play, how I construct my role as manager, and how others construct me in this role, creating the dynamics that emerge between us, particularly when anxiety is triggered by change.

All participants experienced change in relation to their theory of anxiety. These changes occurred as a result of the research process, providing the space to critically reflect together on anxiety. The organisation's endorsement legitimised our exploration of anxiety at work and the underlying assumptions we carried. This resulted in changes to perceptions, where participants practiced less judgement and criticism of colleagues and themselves. This process was successful in emancipating us all in terms of the negative and constraining effect of anxiety at work. We felt safe with each other, and more care of group members emerged. Two participants acknowledged that they noticed anxiety more in their interactions with colleagues and no longer assumed their colleagues' behaviour to be 'difficult or unprofessional'. Participants noticed changes related to 'naming anxiety' as useful in reducing their individual experiences of anxiety.

The research process influenced organisational behaviour. For example, an administration person who greeted staff every morning influenced the participants to respond differently to her polite enquiry about how they were each day. She described how anxiety was communicated to her through the simple exchange of an informal greeting each morning. By the time the fifteenth staff member responded emotionally about how busy they were, her anxiety levels were considerably higher. This was a revelation to everyone in the research group. It led to us all practising a polite reply, that we were well, and to politely ask, how was she? The automatic flood of anxiety communicated previously about our busyness was no longer included once the effect of that communication was understood collectively. This provides an excellent example of how the process made visible an experience of anxiety communicated from one part of the organisation to another. This also revealed understandings about how a subgroup (admin) might change their behaviour to defend or protect against emotion expressed by another organisational subgroup.

Another participant nurse began introducing herself to all new staff from other site locations to assist in reducing feelings of alienation. Talking about anxiety became more acceptable at work:

> it helped with a volunteer who is really anxious. I am really trying to calm her down and say, 'now tell me about how you are feeling'.

The process of the research focused collective attention on the uncomfortable emotions that exist in the organisation, which are usually avoided. These emotions became sources of knowledge about the collective experiences of working in the organisation.

The research process provided evidence for the ways in which critical reflection influenced organisational members' 'theory in use' (Agyris and Schön, 1996), by engaging with current emotional dynamics. The participants used the critical reflection process to challenge the assumptions underlying the theory of anxiety in session one. This resulted in changes to views of anxiety, conflict and changed behaviour. This can be understood as a collective process which promoted organisational learning.

The underlying theory regarding the avoidance of emotion was countered. In the final session, where participants engaged in productive conflict, communication improved. Participants shifted from a position of criticism and blame of others to one where they took both individual and collective responsibility in changing their behaviour. This group decided they wanted critical reflection supervision groups across the service for all staff. The research was presented to the Board, who endorsed and funded the structural changes.

Future directions

The process of critical reflection offers possibilities as a method through which organisations can assist their members with change by building enabling structures through which to attend to the conditions that either inhibit or encourage flexibility. In creating organisational structures through which critical reflection can occur, organisations can assist individual members to reflect on the incidents that become critical for them, to identify their theory of practice and produce the ingredients necessary to examine and evaluate associated practices with the aim of unsettling taken-for-granted assumptions. This opens up possibilities for new ways of knowing to emerge, and a consequent reconstruction of individual theory and practice.

When I was asked to contribute this chapter and to talk about critical reflection and how it has influenced my life, I found this difficult to do. The reason for this is that the learning provided has become integrated into how

I approach life and work. Really learning something that connects theory, practice and values, in the way that critical reflection provides, makes separating out the changes difficult, as they are deeply embedded as a way of knowing for me. I tried hard to think about how I was before critical reflection, and how I am now. Which bits of my way of knowing could I separate out and talk about? In reflecting on this, I realise the benefits that learning in this way can bring. It is a different way of learning that has changed how I manage so that it is now an integrated part of how I think, what I notice and how I approach my work.

I can say that I believe I can positively change how I feel at work. I can have hope about making positive changes at work that positively affect working relationships and bring about a better fit for myself and those with whom I work. As a manager, I engage in cautionary play with pink elephants. I model taking the risk of making them overt; however, making them overt can be a risky thing to do, and if mistimed, managers can get trampled. Trust, timing and careful planning are important to paving the way for critical reflection to be introduced and successfully embedded in an organisation. Inviting colleagues into these practices requires time, patience and preparation so that they might be willing to work with a manager and have hope in the process. A manager needs to ensure there is adequate safety to allow staff to succeed in taking emotional risks to reveal a critical incident in front of their colleagues. This can be anxiety-provoking and a deeply personal disclosure. Hence a cautionary use of power as a theory of practice for me as a manager paves the way for critical reflection and playing with pink elephants.

References

Argyris, C. and Schön, D. (1996) *Organizational Learning II, Theory, Method and Practice*, Reading, MA: Addison-Wesley.
Boyatzis, R.E. (1998). *Transforming Qualitative Information: Thematic Analysis and Code Development*, London: Sage.
Cressey, P., Boud, D. and Docherty, P. (2006) *Productive Reflection at Work: Learning for Change in Organisations*, London: Routledge.
Fook, J. (2002a) *Social Work: Critical Theory and Practice*, London/Thousand Oaks/New Delhi: Sage.
——(2002b) 'Theorizing from practice towards an inclusive approach for social work research', *Qualitative Social Work*, 1(1): 79–95.
Fook, J. and Gardner, F. (2007) *Practising Critical Reflection: A Resource Handbook*, Maidenhead: Open University Press.
Gardner, F. (2006) *Working with Human Service Organisations: Creating Connections for Practice*, Oxford: Oxford University Press.
Garrick, J. and Usher, R. (2000) 'Flexible learning, contemporary work and enterprising selves', *Electronic Journal of Sociology*.
Gould, N. (2000) 'Becoming a learning organisation: a social work example', *Social Work Education*, 19(6).

Gould, N. and Baldwin, M. (eds) (2004) *Social Work, Critical Reflection and the Learning Organisation*, Aldershot: Ashgate.

Hearne, B. (2007) 'Critically reflecting on anxiety as a process that influences organizational learning and change', thesis.

Reynolds, M. and Vince, R. (eds) (2004) *Organizing Reflection*, Aldershot: Ashgate.

Senge, P. (1990) *The Fifth Discipline: The Art and Practice of the Learning Organisation*, Sydney: Random House.

Vince, R. (2001) 'Power and emotion in organizational learning', *Human Relations*, 54(10): 1325–51.

——(2002) 'The impact of emotion on organisational learning', *Human Resource Development International*, 5(1): 73–85.

Section 3
Critical reflection in research

12 The challenges of using critical reflection to develop contextually appropriate social work

Gurid Aga Askeland

Introduction

A few years back I was invited twice to teach an intensive course in critical reflection as part of a new Master's program in social work in Ethiopia. From the students' evaluations, it emerged that they learned about how important context and culture are in social work, as well as about diversity, from hearing about each other's experiences (Askeland and Bradley, 2007; Payne and Askeland, 2008).

Ethiopia has 82 million people and more than seventy-seven ethnic groups, all with their distinct languages and belonging to various religious groups (US Department of State, 2011). Given this diversity, all three of the issues mentioned above could be assumed to be relevant when developing a local professional knowledge base in social work.

With the background from teaching and the students' evaluation, I was encouraged to start a pilot research project using critical reflection to develop contextual social work in Ethiopia. As in many African countries (Mwansa, 2011), Ethiopian students are dependent upon Anglo-American literature. A challenge in this is that ideas of social work developed in these contexts may or may not be directly relevant in Ethiopian contexts. The broad aim of the research project was to develop an understanding of what issues might be specifically identified with Ethiopian social work. Some of the findings have already been reported upon (Askeland et al., 2010).

In this chapter I concentrate on whether critical reflection is a useful research method for developing contextual social work, and what practical challenges are encountered. For the purposes of this study, contextual social work (see Fook, 2002) is understood to be about how social work is practised and conceptualised in relation to the specific and broader context in which it takes place. Context can influence specific meanings and interpretations. In addition, from a postmodern perspective, social work is socially constructed so it may be different depending on the period and the social and historic context (Payne, 2005). Contexts are uncertain, unpredictable and changeable, and vary in size and complexity (Fook, 2002: 143–45).

Organisation and aim of the project

The project was started in 2009 and is still in progress. I knew the PhD students from my former teaching and extended an invitation to them to participate. Some social workers from the field with a Master of Social Work (MSW) degree were also invited through one of the PhD students. Eight participants began the project.

The aim of the project is to develop an understanding of Ethiopian social work directly from the context in which it is practised. The ultimate hope is eventually to produce some locally developed literature which may be used in teaching in the Bachelor of Social Work (BSW) program in Ethiopia and in courses on international social work in western countries.

The first stage of the project took place in February 2009, when I spent three weeks in Ethiopia. The plan was that I would be back in April to follow up with the next stage of the project. However, I was unable to return until a year later, when I spent another three weeks in the country. In between, I had been back for a short visit, and then met up with some of the participants to fix a time that would be suitable for all of us.

Why critical reflection as a research method?

Critical reflection is a method that may be based on different theoretical perspectives. The idea of critical reflection is to reveal underlying individual assumptions that are taken for granted, in order to promote social change. It is both a theory and a practice, and aims at linking changed awareness with changed practice (Fook and Gardner, 2007). It is a bottom-up model to create knowledge from practice. The issues that were presented during the teaching sessions, and what the students reported they had learned from them, inspired me to believe that critical reflection, based on the theoretical framework mentioned in chapter 1, could be a useful research method for discovering issues that would be relevant in developing local social work in Ethiopia. As mentioned above, from a postmodern view, social work is socially constructed and contextual, and may therefore be deconstructed and reconstructed to develop practice theories to fit local communities.

In Ethiopia, with its demographic diversity and its social work students dependent on western professional literature, there might be a huge gap between practice and theory transferred through western literature and by visiting professors. Critical reflection could help to ensure that more contextually relevant knowledge is produced.

Power, oppression and hegemony are important issues in critical theory, which are essential to explore in critical reflection and to become conscious of in order to effect change (Brookfield, 1995, 2009). Revelation of power and oppression embedded in a political regime and bureaucratic system, and its impact on social work, is not the focus of this project. Rather, the idea is to value and integrate how cultural, traditional coping may contribute to developing contextual social work through insight gained via critical reflection. This may lead to emancipation from the hegemony of western professional literature and approaches.

Design of the project

As a research method in the project, we used the critical reflection process as described by Fook and Gardner (2007) and modified it by combining it with focus group interviews.

Critical reflection can be seen as a type of qualitative research method, and is inspired by experiential learning, narrative and an action participatory approach (Askeland, 2011). The idea is that practitioners, by reflecting on their own experiences, will be able to create meaning from their experiences by unearthing fundamental underlying assumptions. There are three important principles for knowledge creation (Fisher, 2005), which I saw as vital to critical reflection in this project, particularly as I come from a different cultural background, and therefore intended to integrate within it.

- Those who are concerned should become involved in deciding the research subject as well as how to analyse the data.
- First-hand experience is highly valued. As an experience takes place in a context, it also has to be understood contextually (Healy, 2000). A close connection between those with direct experience from practice and those who interpret the material will result in more reliable, accurate and less distorted knowledge (Fisher, 2005).
- Knowledge created under these conditions should contribute to emancipation and empowerment.

The critical incident technique was used as a tool for collecting material for critical reflection following the Fook and Gardner model (2007: 76–78). A critical incident is a kind of narrative. Narratives can be told and retold in different ways, which can help in understanding one's own contribution to the development of the situation and creating meaning of experiences. A narrative mirrors the cultural and value system in which the incident has occurred, and is retold.

Focus group interviews can be suitable when exploring new, complex or difficult subjects. I felt this would be a useful adjunct to the critical reflection phase, giving participants a chance to develop collective meanings and knowledge further. In this way, we could develop a shared knowledge base which emerged from the initial personal stories embodied in the critical incidents.

Several researchers and reflexivity

Reflexivity – focusing on the influence of the researcher – becomes imperative in critical reflection because doing research from the position of a neutral outside observer is impossible.

It may be seen as contradictory that I, a white, western social work academic, should come to introduce yet another western model. However, the idea was that my research would not take a 'top-down' approach, but rather that the participants would act as co-researchers in helping each other critically reflect and draw out meaning from their experiences. They would participate in the analysis, and also write up their own critical reflection as book chapters.

The critical reflection design operates with several researchers in different positions, which makes it complex. Three researchers, or groups of researchers, can be distinguished (Askeland, 2008, 2011). The first is the facilitator, who decides upon and introduces the design, and models a critical incident for the participants. During the group sessions, the facilitator may influence the research outcome through her critically reflective questions. Questions are not neutral, but are based on the theoretical foundation, tacit knowledge and experiences of those who pose them. Also, by their mere presence, the facilitator influences the situation and the outcome. There is also some authority and power embedded in a facilitator's position, which may make it difficult fully to meet the principles mentioned above.

The second researcher is the presenter of the critical incident. By opening up to scrutinising their own practice, the presenter becomes a researcher. The topic may vary from presenter to presenter, as they all choose what critical incident they want to focus on. The story they tell is their version of the incident. This story can be considered a text (Taylor and White, 2000), which can be deconstructed and analysed in the same way as an interview (Fook, 1996, 2000). The difference will be that the presenter is also the one who analyses the material and draws out its meaning. What she presents, and also the responses to the posed questions, will influence what outcome she and the group can create from the session. During the critical reflection, the focus will also be on how the presenter as subject contributes to how the critical incident develops, which is culture- and context-bound and depends on personal constructions, social relations and external structures (Fook, 2000: 41).

The final group of researchers in this design would be those I call research assistants or co-researchers. These are the group members who, together with the facilitator, pose critically reflective questions to assist the presenter in going deeper into the material and get a clearer understanding of the situation in order to create new knowledge. Depending on their personal and professional background and experiences, the research assistants may draw out different knowledge from the sessions, which again will influence what common knowledge may be created from the project (Askeland, 2008, 2011).

Stages in the critical reflection

The critical reflection in the project has been divided into three stages. In stage one, I repeated the theoretical basis before the participants each presented an authentic critical incident that they saw as relevant for Ethiopian social work. The presenters critically reflected upon the incidents through critical questions from the other group members and the facilitator. A hand-out exemplified critically reflective questions. During my three week' stay in the country, all the participants presented and reflected on their critical incidents in groups, and the discussions were recorded and transcribed in Ethiopia and distributed to the participants.

Stage two took place a year later. Before my return, the participants were sent material by email about the aim of this stage. As critical reflection is a process, the idea of stage two is to continue the critical reflection to reveal any deeper underlying assumptions, values and beliefs occurring over time, and also to discover whether the process has caused any changes in attitudes and actions. It is also to relabel their personal practice theory which came out of the reflection (see chapter 1). I encouraged the participants to prepare themselves for stage two by going through the transcripts from stage one.

The time gap between the two stages was not intentional. However, it made it necessary, to some degree, to repeat and retell the critical incidents to the group. In this way, the model deviated from Fook and Gardner's (2007), as the model changed from strictly focusing on the reflections of each person presenting in turn, to all group members sharing their experiences and understanding influenced by their various contexts. Consequently, the research design developed into a combination of a critical reflection group, with the focus on the presenter's underlying assumption and mean-ing-making of the critical incident; and a focus group, where the participants contributed with their own experiences, opinions and knowledge and devel-oped a joint understanding of whether the issues raised were of concern in developing local social work. This was concluded by the presenter for-mulating their practice theories as learning they had gained from the critical reflection.

The aim of stage three, a joint analysis seminar, which was intended to follow immediately after stage two, was also communicated to the partici-pants in advance. The aim was to analyse and find relevant and common themes in the critical reflection in order to investigate the overall research questions of the project to develop a contextual social work – what are the issues experienced as specifically relevant to Ethiopia social work, and what are the values behind them? The data to be analysed were the transcripts of the presentations of critical incidents and group exchanges in stages one and two. Participants were asked to prepare for the analysis by going through the transcripts of stage two, which was done parallel to our group work. In the analysis, a narrative model would be used to emphasise the context (Thomassen, 2006). This would provide the basis for writing up the material. The idea has been that each person should write a chapter based on their own critical incident and their critical reflection upon it.

The intention was that, during my three-week stay, we should be able to cover stages two and three and start writing up the material. However, due to cancelling and rescheduling the meetings in stage two, we managed only to start the analysis. The participants then committed themselves to drafting their chapter before we met again, within a certain time limit. This has still to be done.

The emergence of contextual information: the value of critical reflection

During the first stage one participant started his presentation by stating that he was not sure whether his critical incident was relevant for social work. His incident was about his mother having stomach pain and waking up from a bad dream, and then hearing mourning of a dead person at a distance. She immediately interpreted this to mean she was going to die (Askeland et al., 2010). The presenter reflected on how dreams are related to culture and used as a health mechanism. It is part of how people experience reality, and he realised that interpreting dreams had been part of his upbringing. When the group changed into a focus group, the other participants, except for one who had grown up in an urban area, related how they were used to sharing and interpreting their dreams. In stage two, the presenter acknowledged that, through the critical reflection process and group exchanges, he realised that dreams are an issue in social work. It is not for social workers to interpret dreams, as it requires cultural competence, but social workers should recognise how important dreams are in people's lives and for their coping (ibid). His practice theory formulated from his critical reflection was constructivism.

Elders is another issue not commonly related to by western social work literature, with a few exceptions (ibid); this issue is dealt with to some degree in African literature (Osei-Hwedie and Rankopo, 2008). In five out of eight critical incidents presented, elders were mentioned. During the focus groups and analysis, it became clear that elders play a role as counsellors, as negotiators between families, in deciding upon custody of children after divorce, in religious conflicts and in arranging marriages. This shows that social workers should be aware of the elders' roles and might initiate cooperation with them within communities.

Both of these examples demonstrate that critical reflection, combined with focus group interviews, can be used to identify distinctive issues in Ethiopian social work. The participants showed how specific critical incidents from their experience related to what would be seen as important in the culture, issues that might well have been missed altogether or not given sufficient attention from a western perspective.

In stage three, when we had started on the joint analysis of the material, a couple of the participants realised they had several critical incidents they would have liked to present and critically reflect on, and then share in a focus group interview, once they saw the value of the process in relation to developing local social work.

Contextual challenges

Doing research in a developing country, in a different culture from my own, involves challenges related to infrastructure, communication, collecting and analysing the material. These are practical as well as value-based matters, and sometimes constitute two sides of the coin, which complicates the situation.

Commitment

This project has not been the main task for any of us, meaning that it has not always received the necessary priority. With long periods between my visits, the interest understandably seemed to drop. A couple of times I found that, even if we had pre-arranged and agreed upon a time for my return months in advance, appointments with a higher-status project with financial support, which emerged later, had been prioritised without informing me.

The ability to prioritise what is most important at the moment is a practical and value-laden decision, and of course perspectives on this will vary. It is not unusual, even in western settings, that research projects will not be as important to the co-researchers as to the principal researcher. Due to a lack of infrastructure, family matters, responsibility and obligations must take precedence in a non-welfare state. For example, funerals out of town might take several days, causing disruption. Such unpredictability might bring about obstacles to a greater degree than we are used to in western countries.

However, when I have been in Ethiopia, the participants have expressed interest in pursuing the aims of the project. One of those who had been present almost all the time stated at the second stage:

> It becomes more and more interesting every time we meet. What you are doing is a very important investment for the school and I like to work with you.

This might show that there is a connection between commitment, time set aside for the project, and the experienced benefit of the project.

Infrastructure

The social work campus of the Addis Ababa University is based 25 kilometres outside the city centre, and it takes about an hour to get there. A bus service for students and staff runs in the morning and returns in the afternoon. I was mainly dependent on this service. Some of the PhD students have their own cars, while others go by the bus. This means that, having arrived at the campus, one is stuck until the afternoon unless it is possible to get a lift back to town after lunch.

Communication by email has been difficult to keep up. The electricity has been unpredictable. In addition, the internet connection is slow and it takes time to download documents. On my return, some emails from me were found, and some not, when one participant did a search. All the transcripts were done in Ethiopia, and I brought them with me on a memory stick. Before I returned in 2010, I was asked to send all the transcripts in advance as preparation, which I did. However, when I arrived we had to copy the hard copies I brought with me. It has also been difficult to get through on the phone and the connection can often be interrupted.

It is hard to know whether the lack of communication has all to do with infrastructure, or with this project. Some Ethiopian colleagues have indicated that communication is a more general problem; but it has also been hinted to me that exchanges flow more easily when there is money involved, as financial resources are an issue there, as anywhere else.

Time

How we understand and spend time is culture-based and value-laden, and is a complex issue. Behaviour in relation to time reveals how people experience the world around them, and has to be understood contextually. People perceive time consciously, and it has a practical, qualitative and rational aspect. Time is also socially constructed, and there is a link between individual and collective, and between personal and social time.

Although it is impossible to generalise, there are some commonalities that could be applied to African people in contrast to western people (Adjaye, 2002).

According to Adjaye, Africans experience time as multi-level, as a confluence of tradition and modernity, while western people are 'clock-addicted', ruled by the clock in a linear way. Western people are future-oriented and relate to the present as if it is separated from the past, while Africans connect the past and present into the future. Time is also related to change and progress. However, even if the pace might be slower in Africa than in the West, it must not be mistakenly thought that change does not occur (ibid: 214).

Although a meeting time was decided upon by all the participants, the last ones with private cars might show up on the campus 1–1.5 hours after the bus arrived, and might also have to leave earlier, so that the meetings became shorter, and we accomplished less than jointly planned.

A shared understanding of time, where it is possible to interpret each other's messages about appointments, would make social interactions easier. When individual behaviour does not fit the collective understanding, it makes the process even more complex.

I clearly belong to a different time system from the co-researchers with regard to appointments. When western people go by the clock, we might consider people being late or early, as we control, spend, save, waste and run out of time (Payne and Askeland, 2008: 133). Not keeping an appointment might be seen as disrespectful in my culture. Intentionally or unintentionally, it might also be considered to be an exercise of power. Therefore it is necessary to know the context in which relations to time should be interpreted, as well as knowing the individual person's situation and the given infrastructure.

Responding to changing conditions

Sometimes those of us who were present went ahead with the group discussion, although we were aware that not having all members present did
not fit our original research plan. We felt that we had to adapt to what was
possible under the circumstances. At other times, we waited for some time and
then cancelled the meeting, as those present decided that too few participants
had shown up for critical reflection as a group process. Spending hours waiting,
or going back and forth to the campus unable to accomplish anything, would,
in my time system, be considered lost time, so I sometimes found it challenging
to reframe my attitude and learn to adjust. A more western approach might
be to stick to the plan, rather than considering how to adjust to changing
conditions and making explicit what we are doing and why.

Concluding discussion

As mentioned above, this is a pilot project. Nevertheless, according to my
co-researchers, it reinforces that critical reflection in combination with focus
group interviews can bring forward issues of local relevance in developing
contextual social work. The combination of individual critical reflection and
exchanges in focus groups strengthened each other's opinions of the relevance
of the issues.

By deconstructing their concepts of dreams and elders as issues relevant
for local social work, the co-researchers realised that critical reflection, as a
research method incorporating a critical incident technique for collecting
data, can be useful in developing local social work knowledge. These examples
demonstrate that, in a group setting, participants can support, encourage and
facilitate each other to draw out what is distinctive about culture and
how social work practice might be adapted to incorporate this. With the
demography of Ethiopia, where the various ethnic groups have their own
traditions and cultures, critical reflection using critical incidents could
therefore be helpful in focusing on issues relevant for local people.

As a researcher, it is always important to be reflexive, and when doing
research on unfamiliar issues and in cultural settings where the researcher is a
novice, it is particularly required, as it is for me in Ethiopia. In the Ethiopian
setting, I would have to consider myself a cultural novice. Taking into
account all the other challenges, have I, a white, female, western academic,
made a mistake that I was hoping to overcome, by introducing the participants to just another western approach that only in my mind would be
helpful in developing contextual knowledge? Did the method of critical
reflection, which was intended to be a participatory model, partly address
this issue in an effective way? Power is always present and being exercised,
as it was when I modelled critical reflection in the beginning, raising questions
from my own perspective and background.

Clearly, the approach can work. One of the benefits of critical reflection is
having a group, which allows the members to see how their individual

experiences are shared by others and to create a stronger sense of shared knowledge. To become aware of cultural issues that are important in developing local contextual social work is empowering in relation to the hegemonic dominance of western social work.

However, from the challenges we have experienced, I have drawn out some issues for further consideration, and which may assist in better preparation for using such a method in research.

Firstly, in relation to length of time and expected time spent, a limited time for the project might help the participants to be more focused throughout the process. The time gap in this project, while unintentional, has been disruptive. This might be due partly to my residing in another country and not being present all the time throughout the process. Also, when the project is not the main work task, it might be difficult to keep up commitment over time.

Secondly, how to maintain consistent attendance? Or, if this is not possible, how to adapt the project and process? For a critical reflection research process to be reliable, continuity is required. As it happened, particularly in stage two, the various co-researchers attended the group at different times. This made it difficult to build on the work of previous stages, and so made the initial design difficult to adhere to.

Sometimes it may be considered more appropriate to build flexibility into the initial design, feeding back the information from each session to the next.

Thirdly, can common understandings of the theoretical basis and process of critical reflection be sufficient to provide a consistent basis for the research? The co-researchers need to have the same information, otherwise their understanding might differ. With the co-researchers' various attendance, their knowledge and understanding of the theoretical basis and the process also varied. When there are three groups of researchers, as argued above, it is inadequate when not all take part through the whole process, but attend infrequently. The question might be then, what is enough?

Fourthly, it is important to recognise in this approach that, if participants are actually involved as co-researchers, this will mean extra work for them, including preparing by going through the written material and transcripts, and writing up their own experiences. This needs to be acknowledged initially. There also needs to be an up-front need for a commitment to engage with the process.

To conclude, there are clearly benefits in using critical reflection in cultures other than western ones to identify the knowledge and wisdom of practitioners about their particular context. Although there are specific challenges in using critical reflection as a research method in a developing country, such as infrastructure, differences in commitment and/or time may also emerge in other situations. Using critical reflection in this pilot project has, despite the challenges, been promising in unearthing issues that might be of relevance in developing contextual social work further.

References

Adjaye, J.K. (2002) 'Modes of knowing: intellectual and social dimensions of time in Africa', *KronoScope*, 2(2): 199–224.

Askeland, G.A. (2008) *Critical reflection: researching practice*, ESRC funded seminar on critical reflection (Social Work Researcher Development Program), University of Southampton, UK, 23 June.

——(ed.) (2011) *Kritisk refleksjon i sosialt arbeid*, Oslo: Universitetsforlaget.

Askeland, G.A. and Bradley, G. (2007) 'Linking critical reflection and qualitative research on an African social work master's programme', *International Social Work*, 50(5): 671–85.

Askeland, G.A., Mulugeta, E., Ero, D., Negeri, D., Mengsteab, M., Bekele, S. and Alemu, T. (2010) 'Contextual social work in Ethiopia', International Association of Schools of Social Work/International Federation of Social Workers/International Council on Social Work, Hong Kong, 10–14 June.

Brookfield, S. (1995) *Becoming a Critically Reflective Teacher*, San Francisco, CA: Jossey-Bass.

——(2009) 'The concept of critical reflection: promises and contradictions', *European Journal of Social Work*, 12(3): 293–304.

Fisher, M. (2005) 'Knowledge production for social welfare: enhancing the evidence base', in Lang, P. (ed.), *Evidence-Based Social Work: Towards a New Professionalism?* Bern: Peter Lang.

Fook, J. (ed.) (1996) *The Reflective Researcher: Social Workers' Theories of Practice Research*, St Leonards, Australia: Allen & Unwin.

——(2000) 'Deconstructing and reconstructing professional expertise', in Fawcett, B., Featherstone, B., Fook, J. and Rossiter, A. (eds), *Practice Research in Social Work: Postmodern Feminist Perspectives*, London: Routledge.

——(2002) *Social Work: Critical Theory and Practice*, London: Sage.

Fook, J. and Gardner, F. (2007) *Practising Critical Reflection: A Resource Handbook*, Maidenhead: Open University Press.

Healy, K. (2000) *Social Work Practices: Contemporary Perspectives on Change*, London: Sage.

Mwansa, L.-K. (2011) 'Social work in Africa', in Healy, L.M. and Link, R.J. (eds), *Handbook of International Social Work: Human Rights, Development, and the Global Profession*, New York: Oxford University Press.

Osei-Hwedie, K. and Rankopo, M.J. (2008) 'Relevant social work education in Africa: the case of Botswana', in Gray, M., Coates, J. and Bird, M.Y. (eds), *Indigenous Social Work Around the World*, Aldershot: Ashgate.

Payne, M. (2005) *Modern Social Work Theory* (3rd edn), Basingstoke: Palgrave Macmillan.

Payne, M. and Askeland, G.A. (2008) *Globalization and International Social Work: Postmodern Change and Challenges*, Aldershot: Ashgate.

Taylor, C. and White, S. (2000) *Practising Reflexivity in Health and Welfare*, Buckingham: Open University Press.

Thomassen, M. (2006) *Vitenskap, kunnskap og praksis. Innføring i vitenskapsfilosofi for helse-og sosialarbeidere*, Oslo: Gyldendal Akademisk.

US Department of State (2011) 'Background Note: Ethiopia', accessed 23 March 2011, www.state.gov/r/pa/ei/bgn/2859.htm#people

13 Using critical reflection to research spirituality in clinical practice

Janet Allen

Introduction

This chapter discusses the use of critical reflection as a research method for exploring spirituality in my own clinical social work practice with women survivors of sexual trauma. I critically examined my espoused spiritual assumptions and how they impacted my practice using a reflective dialogue process described by Fook (2002). The model I worked with for the purposes of this study was presented in Fook's text *Social Work: Critical Theory and Practice*, and was a precursor to the model developed by Fook and Gardner (2007). My research process involved taking a 'snapshot' of my starting assumptions and then tracing how they evolved and shifted through the course of the critical reflection process. According to Schön (1995), 'knowing in action' involves observing ourselves 'doing' (the practice moment), reflecting on what we notice (critical reflection), providing a description (the transcript), and reflecting on the description (the thematic analysis). This 'knowing-in-action' has the potential to generate new knowledge and theory that can be transferred to new situations, reflected on, and further revised. Fook's (2002) model of critical reflection offered a method for making this tacit process conscious, and introduced an alternative epistemological approach that challenges and reframes traditional ways of knowing and researching by drawing on knowledge that is constructed through everyday experiences.

Throughout this chapter, I explore the use of critical reflection as a research method by detailing some of my methodological struggles and choices, which included navigating the relationship between reflexivity and autoethnography, identifying a priori assumptions, and the formal ethics review process. I also provide some examples of 'findings', or new learnings, that emerged from the inquiry, and conclude with some personal and professional implications regarding the research process and possible directions for future research.

Methodological considerations

Relationship between reflexivity and autoethnography

My research question asked, 'How do my underlying assumptions about spirituality in social work impact my practice with women survivors of sexual trauma?'. While the methodological foundation of the enquiry was clearly qualitative in nature, the question of research design was not as readily evident. Because I was both the sole subject of the research and the researcher, the study fitted within an autoethnographic design. The critically reflective process, therefore, was most appropriately framed as a method of data collection; however, I struggled as a beginning researcher with how to understand the relationship between autoethnography and critically reflective methods.

As conceptualized by Fook (1999, 2002, 2004) and Brookfield (2000), critical reflection is grounded in the traditions of critical social theory and constructivism, includes an analysis of power and domination, and has emancipatory and transformative potential. This process is concerned with the 'story' of what happened and the contributing factors in that storying and meaning-making process, rather than finding the 'truth' or evaluating the situation or the people involved. Similarly, autoethnography uses personal text and acknowledges that stories/narratives can help facilitate change; invites questions about how knowledge, experience, meaning and resistance are expressed and understood; and assumes emotions are important to understanding relationships between self, power and culture (Ellis and Bochner, 2000; Reed-Danahay, 2001; Jones, 2005).

Despite the similarities and congruencies between autoethnography and critical reflection, little has been written regarding the methodological relationship between the two. Since conducting my research in 2006–08, a small but growing body of work has emerged from a number of disciplines, including sociology, education, business and management, psychology, and social work, exploring the relationship between reflexivity and autoethnography. Some scholars, practitioners, and researchers advocate that autoethnography is a means of achieving critical reflexivity (Humphreys, 2005; Jensen-Hart and Williams, 2010). Jensen-Hart and Williams (2010) describe the relationship between reflexivity and autoethnography as a 'natural fit', noting that autoethnography 'facilitates' and 'generates' critical reflexivity. These descriptions suggest that one way of understanding the relationship is that critical reflection is an inevitable product of autoethnography. But could critical reflection be a method in and of itself? Can we conduct autoethnographic research without critical reflection and/or vice versa? Are the two concepts inexorably linked, or best understood as distinct, but related, processes?

McIlveen (2008) proposes 'autoethnography as a qualitative method of reflexive enquiry for narrative research and practice' (p. 14) and explores the concept of 'story' as both data and method. While I chose to differentiate autoethnography as method and critical reflection as data collection for the purposes of my research, McIlveen's argument suggests the potential for challenging a perceived method/data dichotomy, allowing critical reflection to be conceived as both data and method simultaneously.

Identifying a priori assumptions

A second methodological consideration of note was the decision to incorporate the step of identifying consciously held assumptions prior to beginning the critically reflective process. In the critically reflective processes described by Fook (2002, 2004) and Fook et al. (2000), a priori assumptions are not identified before the dialogue sessions – in fact, stage one of the process, the deconstruction phase, aims to identify existing assumptions as well as to allow any new ones to surface. The decision to identify a priori assumptions was based primarily on framing the research question. I found it difficult to develop a specific research question that encompassed the entirety of the critically reflective process. In earlier drafts refining the research question, I framed the purpose of the study as 'What are my underlying assumptions about spirituality in my clinical social work practice with women survivors of sexual trauma?' However, this question spoke directly to identifying assumptions, and I wanted my guiding research question to address the *impact* my assumptions had on my practice. While critical reflection as a method encompasses all of these elements – identification, deconstruction, impact, and reconstruction/revision (see Fook and Gardner, 2007) – it seemed necessary at the time to establish a specific research question that focused on one of these elements. As an attempt to focus more directly on the impact of my own assumptions, I added the step of identifying consciously held assumptions prior to beginning the critically reflective dialogues. Perhaps this step was unnecessary in the use of critical reflection as research method, or perhaps the use of a specific research question is counterintuitive to such a holistic process. Further exploration would be needed to explore these themes in more depth.

As part of the process of defining the terms of the research question, which specifically involved the impact of assumptions and not solely their identification, it was necessary to describe these consciously held starting assumptions. Discussion during the course of a routine supervisory[1] meeting resulted in an impromptu, unstructured interview with my advisor that helped articulate some of my consciously held personal spiritual beliefs, intentions regarding spiritual practice, and understandings of spirituality. Guiding questions posed by my supervisor included 'What are some of your assumptions regarding spirituality?'; 'How do you conceive of spirituality?'; and 'How do you understand spirituality in the context of social work practice?'. This meeting resulted in the identification of nine consciously held assumptions.

I was aware of these initial assumptions as a result of writing, reading, and reflecting on spirituality throughout my life, and of educational, professional, and personal influences and experiences. These initial assumptions relating to spirituality in social work practice were indicative of my thinking and practice approach at the time, and represented my 'beginning' position. The evolution of one of these 'starting' assumptions, namely the assumption that it is necessary to work intentionally with spirituality in practice, is discussed in more detail below.

Ethical considerations

The third methodological issue I discuss here is working with the complex ethical considerations of an autoethnographic, critically reflective study of this nature. Upon beginning this research journey, there was some question/debate among myself, colleagues and advisors as to whether a project based on myself as the sole participant even required a formal ethics review process. However, as the researcher/participant, I was simultaneously subject to both ethics protection and accountability. The ethics proposal (which was approved) focused on potential risks to others and to myself as researcher/participant.

Potential risks to others

The purpose of my research was to examine the process of working with spiritual issues in my own clinical practice. I decided to use only myself as a research participant, because ethically it would be impossible to engage with clients directly as 'subjects'. As the Code of Ethics for the Canadian Association of Social Workers (1994) states: 'A social worker shall not exploit the relationship with a client for personal benefit, gain or gratification' (Clause 4.1, p. 13). In my opinion, asking clients with whom I had a direct therapeutic counselling relationship to participate in my personal research would constitute a violation of professional boundaries and responsibilities that could cause undue harm. Clients' perceptions of how we work together with spirituality in practice were therefore off limits; however, my own perceptions of my practice were an equally valid measure of what was happening in the interactions that took place around spiritual healing.

As the sole research 'subject' in this study, my story of how I construct my practice and consequently the client was the focus of analysis. However, an important ethical consideration when conducting autoethnographic and/ or reflective research is protecting the individuals involved in the stories provided for analysis. The practice moments and the resulting dialogues inevitably involved other 'characters', namely clients, co-workers, supervisors, professors, and/or advisors. To mitigate the possibility of harm, any identifying details respecting these other people involved, however peripherally, were altered or omitted to protect anonymity and confidentiality.

Potential risks to researcher/participant

I approached two partners to assist me in the research who were intimately familiar with Fook's (2002) critically reflective dialogue process and technique.

The roles of the dialogue partners were outlined in a research contract: specifically, that the partners would agree to review the critical practice moments, attend three two-hour dialogue sessions, ask relevant deconstructing and reconstructing questions, and review the resulting transcripts. The contract further clarified my rights as the researcher/participant – the right to withdraw my participation at any time during the process, to refuse to answer any question posed by the dialogue partners, to confidentiality, and to determine dissemination of the results of the research. While the risk to myself as the researcher/participant was minimal, it was still imperative to take steps to mitigate even potential harm. One safety measure put in place was a mandatory check-in between myself and a member of the thesis committee not involved in the dialogue process following each critically reflective dialogue. This committee member was available so I could debrief about the dialogue process, and could also mediate any potential conflicts, in the event the research contract was breached in some way.

'Findings'

Learning: thematic trends

Overall, the reflective learning process was invaluable for exploring contradictions and congruencies regarding the impact of my own assumptions about spiritual and/or religious aspects on my practice with trauma survivors. The most significant learning that came out of the critically reflective dialogue process was the notion that spiritual and/or religious content that emerged in the context of therapeutic practice needed to be 'handled with care'. This enhanced sense of caution around exploring spiritual and/or religious themes in practice extended to the nature of the healing process itself – an assumption that it is a fragile, ephemeral thing and could be easily 'disturbed' by examining spiritual and/or religious beliefs or practices. The idea that spiritual and/or religious values and beliefs are somehow exempt from exploration was connected to dominant individualized discourses around spirituality and religiosity more generally – a commonly heard disclaimer that 'people are entitled to their own beliefs'. In contrast, in my work with trauma survivors, I did not engage that same 'handle with care' approach regarding beliefs about violence, relationships, power, and sexuality. However, spirituality and/or religion seemed off limits, an assumption that has some root in historical professional social work discourses that maintain such themes are 'taboo', oppressive, or irrelevant. As evidenced by more recent attention to spirituality and religion in social work practice, theory, and education, these dominant attitudes seem to be shifting.

This exaggerated sense of caution I identified when working with spiritual and religious themes in practice also had broader implications for my practice more generally. The sense of caution I explored seemed to be mitigated somewhat when working with clients who identified as having marginalized spiritual beliefs. From exploring the practice moments, it was clear that I was more likely to explore/question these more 'alternative' or 'subjugated' belief systems rather than more 'fundamental' or 'conservative' traditions. I connected this trend to assumptions that privileged marginalized spiritualities and denounced religiosity, primarily within Judeo-Christian traditions. In part, I failed to invite exploration due to an underlying belief that disagreement between myself and the client in this area was not okay. It was my understanding that the 'space' or 'airtime' in the session should be filled with clients' spiritual concerns and issues. If my spiritual concerns and issues happen to match, we can share the space; if they do not, clients' issues take precedence. I did not see my spiritual and religious beliefs as important in the counselling process, and operated from an assumption that sharing convergent beliefs would be counterproductive and possibly damaging to the counselling relationship (which, as stated above, I saw as something fragile and precarious). This assumption manifested in practice encounters despite my conscious assertion that appropriate and intentional challenge is necessary and useful in practice interactions. The idea that my spiritual and/or religious beliefs did not matter in the context of counselling interactions extended to an overarching belief that the counselling process itself 'belonged' to the client – not in and of itself a faulty or 'bad' assumption, but one that was not congruent with my espoused understanding of helping that asserts the process (and relationship) are mutually co-created.

Again, while there was nothing inherently 'wrong' with these assumptions, my preference would be to invite exploration of spiritual and religious beliefs in the context of clinical practice. Therefore, in reconstructing my assumptions, it was necessary to acknowledge my capacity consciously to choose between covert disagreement, overt challenge, and neutrality in practice. Now that I am aware that covert disagreement is my 'default' position, I can be clearer about my intention when making that choice. While I still maintain that spiritual practice requires deliberate intention, I would reframe this assumption to reflect that working intentionally with spirituality sometimes requires appropriate challenge.

Reflections on the research process

Several themes stood out when considering my feelings and impressions throughout the course of the research process, which are likely common when sharing any research in an academic context, but seemed amplified in presenting work of such a personal nature. These themes included: feelings of vulnerability, discomfort with not knowing, a perceived need to be assumption-less, expectations about the research process, and concerns regarding the trustworthiness (validity) of this enquiry; they are discussed in more detail below. My experience of these themes represents a source of new knowledge about using critical reflection as a research method.

Vulnerability

Engaging in critical reflection required a high level of vulnerability and personal disclosure. By its very nature, the process seeks to unsettle taken-for-granted assumptions and beliefs, which are often characterized by strong emotional investment (Fook, 2004). Ellis and Bochner point out a similar dynamic respecting autoethnographic enquiry:

> The self-questioning autoethnography demands is extremely difficult. So is confronting things about yourself that are less than flattering ... honest autoethnographic exploration generates a lot of fears and doubts ... then there's the vulnerability of revealing yourself, not being able to take back what you've written or having any control over how readers interpret it.
>
> (Ellis and Bochner, 2000: 738)

The topic of spirituality also felt somewhat 'taboo' and necessitated a high degree of personal disclosure. However, as Fook (2004, 2007) points out, it is in the 'unsettling' that the transformative potential of a new theoretical foundation can emerge.

These vulnerable feelings were particularly strong for me respecting the emotional impact of sharing this information publicly, of holding up my practice for scrutiny and evaluation. Over the course of the research, I identified several assumptions that impacted my practice by encouraging passivity and neutrality, elements that are decidedly uncharacteristic of me in my work and my life. Feelings of vulnerability arose related to how others would interpret this hesitancy and what it might suggest about my abilities as a social worker. At times, this vulnerability resulted in defensiveness, feeling torn between visibility and withdrawal, and confusion, all of which contributed to a lack of focus and motivation. Dealing with these feelings was ultimately an exercise in self-compassion, patience, and creating and utilizing support networks of friends, peers, and colleagues.

Discomfort with not knowing

Connected to these vulnerable feelings was my own discomfort with 'not knowing'. During the dialogues, I struggled to articulate responses to some meaningful questions, and I later felt like I should have been able to answer all questions with ease. After we had finished the data-collection process, I wondered what the dialogue partners thought of me after being exposed in my 'less-than-perfectness' and my 'not-knowingness'. It is not surprising that this discomfort would manifest in a process intended to unsettle taken-for-granted knowledge. I've frequently felt a perception (both within social work circles, and in my life in general) that there is pressure to 'know' all the answers – and not just know them, but to be unequivocally certain about them. Prevailing social, cultural, and professional norms insist we have a clear, concise, and explicit understanding at any given time. My discomfort with 'not knowing' demonstrates just how strongly I have internalized this need for 'certainty', even within a process that is designed to challenge it.

The need to be assumption-less

Another theme that emerged when reflecting on the research process was an assumption that assumptions, in and of themselves, are 'bad' and therefore that I was supposed to strive to be assumption-free (or, at the very least, have the 'right' assumptions). Of course, if I were 'successful' in my pursuit of assumption-less-ness, this would have been a very short study. While I embraced the potential for critical reflection to uncover taken-for-granted perspectives, it was interesting to note a part of myself that was not at all comfortable with the idea that I am inevitably biased and assumption-laden. I neglected the useful, desirable assumptions identified throughout the process and focused primarily on assumptions that were incongruent with my espoused practice principles.

Personally, I found it exhausting continually to dissect experiences and interactions moment-by-moment. The energy and patience this required was something for which I was not fully prepared. In my research process journal, I recorded feeling 'a little annoyed at a process where nothing is taken at face value'. As part of my own spiritual understanding, I believe that we are in a constant state of 'becoming', engaged in a continuous cycle of change and growth, but I also felt the need to achieve a state of equilibrium and rest there, at least for a little while.

I think the act of surfacing assumptions inevitably leads to new contradictions and biases that will appear in another form at some other time. There is always more to learn about one's relationship with the world, with others, with self, and with the divine. However, the never-ending nature of the critical reflection process is not congruent with the predominant professional social work discourses of objectivity and competency-based practice. To gain legitimacy as a social science, social work has promoted 'bias-free' practice. There is a distinct presumption of professional neutrality that I had clearly internalized even as I undertook a study specifically designed to challenge this notion.

Expectations of the research process

Throughout the process, I noted a persistent expectation that critical reflection would unearth some knowledge of which I was previously unaware, although, as I indicated earlier, I was not entirely comfortable when this expectation was fulfilled. This expectation in and of itself implies an internalized positivist understanding of knowledge, that it is fixed, already formed, and intact, and I just had to 'discover' it. Alternatively, critical reflection as developed by Fook (2002) is based in a more subjective understanding of the world that conceptualizes knowledge as constructed, malleable, and transformative. As an example of how this expectation manifested, I deliberately avoided thinking too much about the practice moments prior to the data collection, as I wanted to enter into the dialogues without having done any 'pre-deconstruction'. Reflecting on my cautiousness, I stated that

> Perhaps I carry assumptions about there being a 'right' way to do this, that it is a 'pure' process that I can or will contaminate. This is contrary to my understanding of what critical reflection is for, and could be related to my using it as research in this context – that using it as research requires it to be somehow 'purer' than if I were using it in other ways.

Concerns regarding trustworthiness

I had some concerns about external judgments as to the study's perceived trustworthiness (validity). Although I strongly believe in its value and legitimacy, clearly the research design is outside a traditional positivist framework, which continues to dominate academia. One way these fears manifested was in the tone of the written practice moments themselves, in which I distanced myself from what was happening in the session. There was a conscious effort on my part to maintain some level of formality in academic writing, as if I was trying to validate my work in some imaginary, arbitrary way. In attempting to make my account of the moments more 'objective', I thought on some level that my emotions and investment did not belong. Those internalized expectations around what is valid and what is not are powerful, even in a body of work that is intended to challenge them.

The ethics review process in particular raised doubts as to how others would interpret the 'validity' of my project: fears that it would be rejected by the Ethics Review Board; fears that I had overlooked some fundamental flaw; fears that my own inadequacies would interfere with articulating this complex undertaking. During the proposal-writing phase of the ethics process, I wrote:

> I'm sitting here desperately trying to fit my complex, multi-layered methodology into boxes that are too small, or the wrong shape ... It feels a little bit hopeless, tiring, pointless to go through this exercise in creative knowledge building with a part of me that is uncompromisingly certain that I won't be permitted to pursue the project. 'They're going to reject it', 'they're going to reject it', 'they're going to reject it', replays over and over in my mind.[2]

Furthermore, as if having these pervasive and, at times, paralyzing doubts was not enough, I noted feelings of 'embarrassment that I have these doubts, these gaps in my consciousness'. These doubts demonstrated the entrenched internalization of positivist assertions that use of self is not empirically sound and that so-called 'subjective' knowledge is inherently invalid.

Consistent reminders from friends, colleagues, supervisors, and committee members as to the validity of socially constructed knowledge and reflexive meaning-making were an essential source of support and, in my opinion, paramount for anyone undertaking such a research process.

Suggested directions for future research

Critical reflection as research method

There were several choices made in applying Fook's (2002) critically reflective technique in this adaptation of its use as research method that are important to explore further. Firstly, it would be useful to consider the impact of identifying initial assumptions independent of the critically reflective dialogues themselves. While appropriate for the purposes of this enquiry due to the nature of the research question, the value or role of this step needs to be explored further in developing critical reflection as a research method. Secondly, I made the decision to use three distinct practice moments for analysis, which was based on an intuitive sense of the volume of data required to reach a saturation point. Experimenting with the number of practice encounters used for analysis in such enquiries would provide useful information about critical reflection as a research process. Thirdly, due to scheduling challenges, there was an unavoidable six-week gap in between the first dialogue session and the subsequent sessions. The dialogue partners and I agreed to conduct the remaining two sessions on the same day, also as a scheduling convenience. Without a source of comparison, it is not practical to speculate on the effect this six-week gap may have had on the data. The importance of consistent and systematic data collection respecting critically reflective methods needs to be considered in more depth.

Critical–spiritual reflective processes

There are aspects of dialogic reflexivity that are inherently spiritual and critical, introducing an emerging process of 'critical–spiritual reflection'. As individuals and professionals, social workers are influenced by religious and/or spiritual discourses (Todd, 2004). Accordingly, it is necessary to deconstruct such discourses and examine their influences on identity and the profession of social work itself. This deconstruction is important for addressing spirituality in the context of critical social work with a view to connecting spirituality, social justice issues, and structural inequalities in society.

One suggestion for future research respecting critical–spiritual reflection in practice is to explore different ways of incorporating the method with other social workers in the dialogues around spirituality in practice. Fook (2004) points out that dialogue sessions can be facilitated in groups of mutually invested people, such as clients, social work practitioners, or students. For instance, Canda (2006) suggests exploring inter-religious dialogues and advocates pursuing interdisciplinary research in the field of spirituality and health. My research provides an example of how critical reflection can be used to initiate dialogue around practitioners' spiritual beliefs, which could also be adapted to help social work students explore spiritual assumptions in an academic context.

My study focused on critical–spiritual reflection in clinical practice, but critical reflection could also be applied to examining spirituality in other social work practice contexts, such as case management, and community organizing and development.[3] Such research would be particularly useful for debunking myths of shared subjectivity or collective consciousness that contribute to the marginalization of difference, and also for examining core values and goals in collectives (Shragge, 2003).

Additionally, I would suggest that critically–spiritually reflective work connects, even in a small way, Freire's (1972) link between deepening con-sciousness and humanization: 'The pursuit of full humanity, however, cannot be carried out in isolation or individualism, but only in fellowship and solidarity' (p. 73). The process of taking apart the 'taken-for-granteds' in the context of research was a profound (and very public!) acknowledgement of my own humanness – an acknowledgement that I feel is essential for realizing the transformative potential of critically reflective learning.

Notes

1 This research was undertaken in fulfillment of a Master's of Social Work degree at Dalhousie University, and was therefore supervised.
2 Fortunately these fears proved unfounded as the ethics proposal for this research was approved upon initial review and required no revisions.
3 See Damianakis (2006) and Todd (2004) for research that explores the spiritual dimensions of organizational change within the context of feminist organizing.

References

Brookfield, S.D. (2000) 'The concept of critically reflective practice', in Wilson, A.L. and Hayes, E.R. (eds), *Handbook of Adult and Continuing Education*, San Francisco: Jossey-Bass, 33–49.
Canda, E.R. (2006) 'Spiritual connection in social work: boundary violations and transcendence', keynote address delivered at the First North American Conference on Spirituality and Social Work, 25–27 May, University of Waterloo, Ontario.
Damianakis, T. (2006) 'Seeking the spiritual in anti-oppressive organizational change', *Critical Social Work*, 7(1).
Ellis, C. and Bochner, A.P. (2000) 'Autoethnography, personal narrative, reflexivity: research as subject', in Denzin, N.K. and Lincoln, Y.S. (eds), *Handbook of Qualitative Research* (2nd edn), Thousand Oaks: Sage, 733–68.
Fook, J. (1999) 'Reflexivity as method', in Daly, J., Kellehear, A. and Willis, E. (eds), *Annual Review of Health Social Sciences*, 9: 11–20.
——(2002) 'New ways of knowing', in Fook, J. (ed.), *Social Work: Critical Theory and Practice*, London: Sage.

——(2004) 'Critical reflection and transformative possibilities', in Davies, L. and Leonard, P. (eds), *Social Work in a Corporate Era: Practices of Power and Resistance*, Aldershot: Ashgate, 28–42.

——(2007) 'Reflective practice and critical reflection', in Lishman, J. (ed.), *Handbook for Practice Learning in Social Work and Social Care* (2nd edn), London: Jessica Kingsley, 363–75.

Fook, J. and Gardner, F. (2007) *Practising Critical Reflection: A Resource Handbook*, Maidenhead: Open University Press.

Fook, J., Ryan, M. and Hawkins, L. (2000) *Professional Expertise: Practice, Theory and Education for Working in Uncertainty*, London: Whiting & Birch.

Freire, P. (1972) *Pedagogy of the Oppressed*, New York: Herder & Herder.

Humphreys, M. (2005) 'Getting personal: reflexivity and autoethnographic vignettes', *Qualitative Inquiry*, 11(6): 840–60.

Jensen-Hart, S. and Williams, D.J. (2010) 'Blending voices: autoethnography as a vehicle for critical reflection in social work', *Journal of Teaching and Learning in Social Work*, 30: 450–67.

Jones, S.H. (2005) 'Autoethnography: making the personal political', in Denzin, N.K. and Lincoln, Y.S. (eds), *Handbook of Qualitative Research* (3rd edn), Thousand Oaks: Sage, 763–91.

McIlveen, P. (2008) 'Autoethnography as a method for reflexive research and practice in vocational psychology', *Australian Journal of Career Development*, 17(2): 13–20.

Reed-Danahay, D. (2001) 'Autobiography, intimacy and ethnography', in Atkinson, P., Coffey, A., Delamont, S., Lofland, J. and Lofland, L. (eds), *Handbook of Ethnography*, London: Sage, 407–25.

Schön, D.A. (1995) 'The new scholarship requires a new epistemology', *Change*, 27(6): 26–35.

Shragge, E. (2003) 'Towards a conclusion: community organizing and social change', in *Activism and Social Change: Lessons for Community and Local Organizing*, Peterborough, ON: Broadview Press, 187–207.

Todd, S. (2004) 'Feminist community organizing: the spectre of the sacred and the secular', *Currents: New Scholarship in the Human Services*, 3(1), http://wcmprod2.ucalgary.ca/currents/files/currents/v3n1_todd.pdf

14 Some methodological and ethical tensions in using critical reflection as a research methodology

Christine Morley[1]

Introduction

This chapter outlines some of the methodological and ethical issues inherent in using Fook and Gardner's (2007) model of critical reflection as a research methodology. Many pedagogical issues related to using critical reflection as a learning tool in the context of education are well theorised and documented in the literature. These include: the educator taking a leadership role in fostering critical reflection as part of transformative learning (Brookfield, 2005: 352; Giroux, 2011: 3); the politics of both the educator and the learner contributing to a co-construction of new knowledge (Brookfield, 2005: 358); and the power relations between the educator facilitating the critical reflection and the learner engaging in it (Brookfield, 2005: 354; Giroux, 2011: 5). However, such issues are less well articulated in relation to using critical reflection as a tool of inquiry in the context of research. This chapter discusses these tensions, and presents my reflections about conducting critically reflective research with social work practitioners to explore the possibilities to work towards changing the legal response to sexual assault. I also explore conducting this type of research in organisational settings such as universities, and discuss the challenges this can present as dominant, objectivist ways of knowing are often privileged within these contexts (Meinert et al., 2000). I ultimately argue that Fook and Gardner's (2007) model of critical reflection model offers a rigorous and ethical method of inquiry.

The research project involved working with six experienced sexual assault practitioners who were employed as counsellor/advocates.[2] All participants were concerned that their work with victims/survivors had become dominated by responding to the failures of the legal system to deliver justice. This secondary, systemic abuse perpetrated by the legal system was producing a strong sense of fatalism in practitioners. Consequently, all participants initially expressed a strong sense of powerlessness.

Critical reflection

The methodology I used in this project was based on Fook's (2002) model of critical reflection, which bears some similarities to the more recent iteration developed by Fook and Gardner (2007). These models of critical reflection involve a process of elucidating how the discourses we use to understand and construct our world are instilled with dominant power relations and practices (Fook, 2002). They are based on the premise that 'the surfacing of assumptions held by individual people about their social worlds may ultimately lead to a capacity to change the ways that people act in relation to their social contexts' (Fook and Gardner, 2007: 14). Therefore I used Fook (2002) because it held the potential to create different ways to think about the problem of sexual assault counsellor/advocates not feeling that they had the agency to challenge and change the legal response to sexual assault.

I adapted this model of critical reflection to apply it as a research methodology by gathering and analysing six case studies about counsellor/advocates' practice (Morley, 2008, 2011b). These narratives were critical incidents from participants' practice that captured their perceptions of the main problems with the legal system and the barriers they saw to creating change. Analysing cycles of thinking embedded with critical incidents is fruitful, as they often indicate more generic responses (Brookfield, 2005). When using critical incidents to research practice, participants examined their construction of the story, and through immersion in the critical reflection process, created the possibility to re-author their story along more empowering lines which developed new directions for change (Fook, 2002: 99; Napier and Fook, 2000: 10).

Given that this approach to critical reflection involves a two-stage process (Fook and Gardner, 2007), I met with each participant twice. Each interview took between 60 and 90 minutes to complete. The first stage was to hear their story and begin to deconstruct it with them. Deconstruction involves identifying hidden values and assumptions in our thinking and action that are problematic for, or contrary to, our intended or espoused practice (Fook and Gardner, 2007; Taylor and White, 2000; Fook, 2002). I was therefore asking questions to unearth unhelpful interpretations that contributed to practitioners' sense of powerlessness. For example, some of the deconstruction questions included the following:

- What do you think are the implications for you, and for your practice, if you see your service users, and yourself, as utterly powerless?
- How might positioning yourself in opposition to the police, who you see as having all the power, lead you to feel more disempowered?
- Who benefits from this cycle of thinking?
- How does this thinking compare with your espoused intention to support and advocate for victims/survivors?

The second stage was to assist participants to reconstruct their story, which involved generating new ways of thinking and related practices that provide fresh strategies to respond to the difficulties they described (Fook, 2002; Fook and Gardner, 2007). This involved assisting participants to reinterpret their stories in ways that generated a hopefulness for change and practical agency to respond. For example, some of the reconstruction questions included the following.

- How does that notion that you can exercise power free you to practise differently with the police?
- Can you think about some exceptions to your narrative that construct the service users as totally powerless in every context?
- Can you share some examples when either you and/or your service users displayed acts of resistance?
- How does this change your thinking about practice?

Theoretical ideas from critical social work that draw on the postmodern notion of multiple truths were used to assist the participants to consider their story as one possible construction (among many possible constructions). This enabled participants to recognise that their personal interpretation of their critical incident was created through their own participation in discourse (Seidman, 2004). This challenged the initial positioning of their account as 'reality', or *the* truth (Rossiter, 2005). This theoretical stance makes visible the possibility of multiple interpretations of the same story, which created the 'conceptual space' (Rossiter, 2005: 1) for participants to develop innovative ways to re-think the problems with the legal response to sexual assault, and how they positioned themselves in relation to barriers to change. I was therefore hoping to engage practitioners in a critically reflective process that connected them with a sense of power and agency.

Ethical and methodological issues

The researcher as facilitator of transformative learning

Within the context of education, deep, transformative learning (Ramsden, 1998) enables the process of critical reflection to create and envision change possibilities. As Brookfield (2005: 354) explains:

> Teaching in a manner informed by critical theory is ... inherently political ... It is political because it makes no pretense of neutrality, though it embraces self-criticism. It is political because it is highly directive ... This political emphasis is scattered throughout the history of critical theory.

However, when using critical reflection as a research methodology, this same political potential implicates researchers in trying to change their participants through the research process, which can be identified as an ethical problem by some researchers. As with critical education, most social research results in some form of intervention with the people we are researching (Sarantakos, 2005), whether or not the researcher/s are conscious and intentional about this aspect of their research. However, at times I felt very aware of the ethical and methodological tensions for myself as a researcher, engaged in purposely trying to 'transform' my participants.

This goal differs radically from approaches to research that are predicated on the assumptions of traditional, objectivist or realist paradigms, and reflects the 'paradigm wars' (Loftus et al., 2011: 3) that characterise debates about the nature of knowledge, 'truth', 'reality' and meaning (see for example Meinert et al., 2000; Sarantakos, 2005; Morris, 2006; Humphries, 2008). From an objectivist view, it is believed possible and essential to separate the object from the subject and the researcher from the research participants, processes and outcomes (Meinert et al., 2000; Sarantakos, 2005). This belief in the possibility of objective knowledge supports the ontology that a true knowledge about reality is possible (Meinert et al., 2000). Therefore, from this standpoint, data should be collected through objective and external means in order to find the truth about social phenomena (Humphries, 2008; Loftus et al., 2011), but certainly not to form a critically reflective view of participants' experiences in order to work with them to deconstruct, and then reconstruct, the knowledge that we were collaboratively developing from the research process, as we were in this project.

Continuing to violate the ethics, ontology and epistemology of objectivist research, I was involved not only in facilitating transformational learning in my research participants, but also in doing this in a way in which I thought they should be transformed – in line with the emancipatory goals and values of a critical social work approach (Fook, 2002; Allan et al., 2009), critical pedagogical approaches (Giroux, 2011), and critical and constructivist research paradigms (Morris, 2006; Humphries, 2008).

One participant chose to describe an incident where she felt disempowered and disappointed in her practice, because she believed at the time that she didn't have the right or the power to challenge police who dismissed a disclosure of sexual assault made by a victim/survivor who had an intellectual disability. In this situation, my role in the critical reflection research process was not simply to gather information and document her story, as an objectivist approach to research would (Arnd-Caddigan and Pozzuto, 2006; Loftus et al., 2011), but to aim to assist this practitioner to recognise the advocacy component of her role, challenge her assumptions about being powerless, and connect her with a sense of agency that makes possible the challenging of inappropriate, unethical behaviours by police (Morley, 2011a).

An objectivist position would be troubled by the researcher becoming the main tool of data generation, as I did in this project. Engaging in a series of critically reflective questions (Fook, 2002: 92–101; Fook and Gardner, 2007: 75–76) to elucidate constructions that improve participants' practice may well be viewed as 'contaminating' the data from an objectivist perspective (Arnd-Caddigan and Pozzuto, 2006).

However, in an educational setting, Giroux (2011: 3) would regard this pedagogical practice as necessary for 'creating the conditions for producing citizens who are critical, self-reflective, knowledgeable, and willing to make moral judgments and act in socially responsible way[s]'. Some researchers similarly argue that the role of research should be to 'understand social reality in ways that [will] provide insights towards the creation of a more emancipatory society' (Popkewitz, cited in Goodman, 1998). Loftus et al. (2011: 5, citing Higgs and Titchen, 2007) argue that 'if research is to be truly useful and move our understandings forward then it … needs to be creative and transformative'.

However, by facilitating a critically reflective conversation with this participant, I was implicated in the sort of knowledge that we produced, and ultimately the ways in which our discussion influenced the outcomes of the research. This also extended to how I assembled and presented the data.

During my interactions with this participant, I felt conscious of privileging particular narratives and making certain assumptions about how practice *should* be. When this practitioner discussed her hesitation to challenge the police about their inappropriate conduct towards the service user, my work with her, and the reflective questions that I posed, inhered a judgment that she *should* have challenged them. From a critical perspective in the context of adult learning, this may be considered an example of educator leadership (Giroux, 2011: 5). I was not a dispassionate, passive gatherer of information, but an active participant in the construction of the sort of knowledge produced (Powell, 2002; Sarantakos, 2005; Loftus et al., 2011). As part of a dialogical process, I was also changed and transformed by the critical reflection process. My position in this process and the constructions that I formed throughout were frequently altered as I was often challenged to re-evaluate and shift my thinking in light of the dialogue I was having with the participants and what they brought to the process.

Within adult educational discourses, assuming this fluid type of role to foster critical reflection in learners is regarded as an important and appropriate part of the transformative learning process (Brookfield, 2005; Giroux, 2011). However, within objectivist research discourses, my positioning in the research as a co-constructor of knowledge meant that I had biased the research (Humphries, 2008: 10) by influencing the research participants to follow particular pathways – the pathways that I felt would be most beneficial – based on my critical social work theoretical lens (Fook, 2002; Allan et al., 2009). This is a dilemma created by the fundamental epistemological differences between objectivist-based approaches to research that claim to find knowledge through objective research processes (Arnd-Caddigan and Pozzuto, 2006), and a critically reflective epistemological position where the researcher is entirely transparent about their responsibilities to engage in research that produces rather than finds knowledge (Meinert et al., 2000; Fook and Gardner, 2007; Morley, 2008).

Whilst an objectivist view considers my positioning in the research as a fundamental flaw, critical reflection, with its goal of emancipatory transformative learning and reconstruction (Fook, 2004), considers my reflexive positioning and influence over the production of data as a strength that contributes to greater depth and richer outcomes (White, 2001; Powell, 2002; Humphries, 2008: 29–30). From an objectivist standpoint, that which is knowable must exist independently of the knower (Arnd-Caddigan and Pozzuto, 2006). However, this objectivist position would simply serve to reinforce the powerlessness of the practitioners by leaving the data/stories that they provide untouched and intact. From the objectivist perspective, the telling of the story is its end. In contrast, from a critically reflective perspective, the initial telling of the story is just the beginning of a process that will evolve as the story is told and re-told in different ways, emphasising different aspects and including new information. As Loftus et al. (2011: 7) explain, 'The task of creative approaches to researching living practices is to reveal and symbolically re-present them ... The acceptance of multiple perspectives welcomes creative and diverse ways of collecting, re-presenting and interpreting data.' Critical reflection therefore positions participants' identities as 'evolving construction[s] that manifest ... during conversations' (Sands, 1996: 177). Therefore, as the person to whom the stories were being told, I was implicated in the construction of the participants' narratives (Frost, 2006). Whilst the need to respect and validate participants' experiences was clear, I also felt I had an ethical responsibility to challenge unhelpful assumptions that I perceived were exacerbating participants' sense of powerlessness. This is appropriate because 'In qualitative research we need to be quite clear about the purpose of the research and creatively come up with an interpretation that best suits that purpose' (Loftus et al., 2011). Deconstruction and reconstruction were therefore employed to assist the participants to form alternative understandings that were potentially more empowering and enabling, as critically reflective researchers have a responsibility to contribute to more emancipatory outcomes (Fook, 2002; Fook and Gardner, 2007).

Critical reflection as ethical research

From a critical social work perspective, it could be considered unethical to avoid participating in the research in this way (Humphries, 2008: 19). This was highlighted for me recently when, in carrying out a number of small research projects related to the learning and teaching of critical reflection, the ethics committee within the university would not allow me, as the educator and researcher, to interview graduates about their experiences of critical pedagogy. Through the privileging of objectivist understandings of research, distance is valorised over familiarity (Arnd-Caddigan and Pozzuto, 2006). Consequently, it was argued that my proposed participation in the research to conduct a focus group would be unethical because of the teaching role I had previously occupied. It transpired that a colleague who had not been involved with teaching critical reflection to the graduates concerned conducted the focus group instead. The colleague did an exemplary job; however, because he was not an insider (White, 2001) to the research process, he asked the series of questions that I prepared, but was not able to engage in a genuine dialogue with the graduates, which meant their contribution to the research was not reciprocated.

Taking a critically reflective stance, this presented an ethical issue for me as I saw it as a wasted opportunity to enhance and reinforce the graduates' learning. For example, one of the questions asked about the barriers in the workplace to engaging in critically reflective practice. The graduates recited the usual reasons, such as being 'too busy' and 'not having enough time to reflect'. In listening to the recording of this focus group after its completion, I felt the students could have benefited from having the opportunity to deconstruct such assumptions, particularly when their implications may hold serious limitations for the practice that they take out into the field. In this way, the methodological policing of critical reflection from an unstated, objectivist position actually deprived graduates of learning opportunities that would have otherwise been provided by using critical reflection as the research method. In following the canons of the ethics committee that required the interviewer to be distant, external and removed from the graduates in order to 'protect' them, the insights generated by the research were artificially and unnecessarily limited.

Reflexivity

Whilst all research paradigms quite legitimately raise questions about how a researcher can ensure that she or he is conducting the research in an ethical manner, when considering fostering transformation in the research participants along critical and emancipatory lines, it is critically reflective methodologies that provide the intellectual space to institute mechanisms of reflexive rigour in ways that are both transparent and accountable (Morley, 2008). For the research with sexual assault practitioners, this required me to engage in a parallel critically reflective process that ensured my practice as researcher was consistent with my espoused goals of critical social work. This theoretical perspective provides 'a broader framework for understanding what critical reflection can and should help achieve' (Fook, 2004: 20), particularly in the context of professional learning in social work. Facilitation of critical reflection by an educator or by a researcher is therefore not a random process or one determined by the researcher's values without responsibility. The theoretical frameworks that underpin critical reflection provide a rigorous and ethical form of accountability (Morley, 2008).

Reflexivity – the impact and influence of the researcher, and the importance of self-reflection and critique (Powell, 2002; Humphries, 2008) – is therefore a central consideration in evaluating the worth of research that uses critical reflection as a methodology (Fook, 1999). Reflexivity is 'the ability to locate oneself squarely within a situation, to know and to take into account the influence of personal interpretation, position and action within a specific context' (Fook, 2000: 17, cited in Humphries, 2008: 28).

Power relations between researcher and researched

Furthermore, the practice of working with participants to construct alternative understandings of situations by which they initially felt disempowered was scrutinised and problematised by the critically reflective methodology. For example, for at least one participant, the process of destabilising particular assumptions was very challenging. Whilst she was able to engage in the critical reflection process to some degree, she paradoxically commented that she was happy with her original interpretation and saw its limitations as a compromise, even though she felt 'stuck' in terms of thinking about creative practice responses. For this participant, innovative reconstructions of her practice were less forthcoming than for some of the other participants, but this certainly did not mean that I imposed my perspective about how I thought her critical incident could be reconstructed. In keeping with the emancipatory aims of critical social work (Allan et al., 2009), I consciously resisted prescribing the particular constructions that I would have liked to see privileged. Consistent with the theoretical frameworks underpinning critical reflection, my role in working with this participant, both as critically reflective researcher and as facilitator of transformative learning and practice, took the form of discussing various constructions and options and sharing different theoretical viewpoints, but ultimately respecting her position and her interpretations of reality (Fook and Morley, 2005).

This invites consideration of the ethical dimensions of the research in terms of the power relations between researcher and researched. In objectivist research, the researcher is seen as removed from the research process (Meinert et al., 2000; Humphries, 2008). In contrast, some acknowledge that 'subjectivity is present in all research' and consider that 'subjective experience is itself a source of valuable insights' (Loftus et al., 2011). In addition, a critical social work perspective considers this understanding to create artificial, binary oppositional and hierarchical power relations between researcher and research participants (Fook, 2002). In drawing on critical postmodern commitments, I did not wish to reproduce these power relations by maintaining a pretence that it was possible for me to engage in this research whilst remaining independent and external.

One of the ways in which I attempted to resist this artificial dichotomous construction was to simultaneously engage in the research as a participant, and share my critical reflection in my practice with the other participants. This enabled me to model the courage and humility required to engage in the process of critical reflection as a learning experience in order to improve practice. Through sharing my reflection and learning, I could demonstrate, for example, that we are all, at times, affected by dominant discourses. Positioning myself as a research participant also provided the opportunity for me to make reference to particular themes inherent in my practice scenario, so that participants could identify similar themes in their own practice. For example, the critical incident on which I reflected involved my participation in adversarial and oppositional power relations with a particular detective who I perceived as breaching the police code of conduct by bullying the service user I was supporting (Morley, 2009). Other participants were able to recognise the unintended consequences of this conflict for my practice, and able to see parallels about the limiting effects for their practice where they, too, had been drawn into conflict that they felt disempowered them.

The decision to include my critical reflection with the other participants was important in contributing to a respectful, non-judgemental, open and trusting culture in which to critically reflect. This normalised the learning from critical reflection and freed participants to resist the pressures to always be 'right' or be seen to be doing 'best practice', instead genuinely to engage in a critical reflection process that would enhance their under-standing, performance and agency in the context of critical social work goals (Fook, 2002). These conditions have been identified as a central component of the environment required for critical reflection in education (Fook, 2004; Gardner et al., 2006; Fook and Gardner, 2007), and the aforementioned project demonstrates that this is equally applicable when using critical reflection in research.

Outcomes of the research

Had I used objectivist or realist approaches, the research would have been restricted to attempts at documenting the participants' narratives independently of myself, to discover 'absolute truth' consisting of 'verifiable facts' (Meinert et al., 2000: 46) in the most objective manner possible with 'accurate measurements' that enable 'cause/effect mechanisms to be explained' (Loftus et al., 2011: 3). This would have maintained the participants' initial sense of hopelessness and powerlessness. Conversely, using critical reflection to research the problem of practitioners' sense of powerlessness produced very different, and arguably far more useful, outcomes than what an objectivist approach would have 'found'.

The process of using critical reflection as a methodology for research was both a humbling and an emancipatory experience for myself and the other participants. Examining the contributions that our thinking had made to particular discourses that were unhelpful for our practice and operating contrary to our goals was, at times, very difficult. However, realising we had the capacity to change our construction of the problem, and our response in relation to it, was thoroughly liberating.

All participants reported that they had benefited from the critical reflection process and enjoyed their participation in it, which parallels other observa-tions about using critical reflection (Fook, 2004: 23). Most practitioners understood and embraced the critical reflection processes, began to pre-empt my questions part way through our interviews, and commenced generating their own examples of reconstructed practice. This enabled the outcomes that emerged to be much more instructive for emancipatory change-orientated practice than I could have anticipated, or would have been able to achieve without their contributions to the research.

One participant, for example, initially described watching in horror as a court process unfolded that completely undermined and invalidated the testimony of the victim/survivor she was supporting. Through a series of critically reflective questions that aimed to reconstruct alternative interpretations of her capacity to use power by participating in the construction of discourse (Fook, 2002; Fook and Gardner, 2007: 108; Smith, 2008: 32–34), this participant came to the realisation that she could ask the prosecution to subpoena her as an expert witness. This created the opportunity for her to resist the social mythology that was undermining the credibility of the victim/survivor's testimony in court and replace this with a more informed perspective.

Another participant, who initially described feeling excluded by the operations of elite legal personnel, realised through being asked similar questions to the former participant, such as: 'How does the postmodern notion that power can be exercised free you to think about quite differently about your initial construction of powerlessness?', that she could organise a meeting and invite the key people with whom she wanted to consult.

The creation of these reconstructed discourses enabled a much more proactive response on the part of the participants than their original constructions had allowed. Critical reflection facilitated the reconstruction of their roles in ways that were more affirming of the value of their work and more appreciative of their power and agency to work towards change. Hence, using critical reflection as a research methodology resisted participants' initial sense of powerlessness and fatalism, and created transformative possibilities. Whilst this capacity of critical reflection has been widely known for some time when used as a model of education (Fook, 2004: 24), it is useful to understand how these same goals can be achieved through using critical reflection as a research methodology.

Conclusion

This paper has explored using critical reflection as a method of inquiry in research. It has consequently raised some important philosophical considerations about the dominantly constructed dualisms between the researcher and the researched; the relationship between the knower and the known; objectivity versus reflexivity; distance versus familiarity; the finding of data rather than the production of knowledge; and the insider versus outsider positioning of the researcher. It is hoped that this exploration has highlighted how limited and limiting the dominant, objectivist ways of knowing can be for social research, which has a much broader potential to contribute towards emancipatory change. Such artificial dichotomies that are perpetuated by the dominant view also raise questions about the ethical versus the unethical conduct of research, as if there is a universal truth about ethical standards.

Through exploration of the ethical and methodological issues involved in using critical reflection as a research methodology, such as the researcher fostering transformative learning as part of the research; the politics of both researcher and researched contributing to a co-construction of new knowledge; and the power relations between researcher and research participants, I hope to have demonstrated how the dominant objectivist paradigm denies that our constructions of ethical practice are created by various discourses and the power invested in them, and that these discourses shift and change depending upon the epistemological framework in which the research is located and judged. Ultimately, I have argued that critical reflection offers a rigorous and ethical methodology for social research that intends to contribute to transformative learning and emancipatory aims.

Notes

1 Acknowledgement: thank you to Dr Phillip Ablett, Lecturer in Sociology at the University of the Sunshine Coast, who generously contributed to the discussion and ideas that informed this chapter.
2 This term is used to refer to the practitioners who work in Centres Against Sexual Assault in Victoria, Australia. These practitioners are usually social workers or qualified professionals in related disciplines.

References

Allan, J., Pease, B. and Briskman, L. (eds) (2009) 'Developing feminist practices', in *Critical Social Work: An Introduction to Theories and Practices*, Crows Nest, NSW: Allen & Unwin.

Arnd-Caddigan, M. and Pozzuto, R. (2006) 'Truth in our time', *Qualitative Social Work*, 5(4): 423–40.

Brookfield, S. (2005) *The Power of Critical Theory for Adult Learning and Teaching*, Maidenhead: Open University Press.

Fook, J. (1999) 'Reflexivity as Method', *Annual Review of Health Social Sciences*, vol 9: 11–20.

——(2000) 'Deconstructing and reconstructing professional expertise', in Fawcett, B., Featherstone, B., Fook, J. and Rossiter, A. (eds), *Practice and Research in Social Work: Postmodern and Feminist Perspectives*, London: Routledge.

——(2002) *Critical Social Work*, London: Sage.

——(2004) 'Critical reflection and transformative possibilities', in Davies, L. and Leonard, P. (eds), *Social Work in a Corporate Era: Practices of Power and Resistance*, Aldershot: Ashgate, 16–30.

Fook, J. and Gardner, F. (2007) *Practising Critical Reflection: A Resource Handbook*, Maidenhead: Open University Press.

Fook, J. and Morley, C. (2005) 'Empowerment: a contextual perspective', in Hick, S., Fook, J. and Pozzuto, R. (eds), *Social Work: A Critical Turn*, Toronto: Thompson, 67–85.

Frost, S. (2006) 'Recasting individual practice through reflection on narratives', in White, S., Fook, J. and Gardner, F. (eds), *Critical Reflection in Health and Social Care*, Maidenhead: Open University Press, 107–17.

Gardner, F., Fook, J. and White, S. (2006) 'Critical reflection: possibilities for developing effectiveness in conditions of uncertainty', in White, S., Fook, J. and Gardner, F. (eds), *Critical Reflection in Health and Social Care*, Maidenhead: Open University Press, 228–40.

Giroux, H. (2011) *On Critical Pedagogy*, New York: Continuum.

Goodman, J. (1998) 'Ideology and critical ethnography', in Smyth, J. and Shacklock, G. (eds), *Being Reflexive and Critical in Educational and Social Research*, London: Falmer Press, 50–66.

Higgs, J. and Titchen, A. (2007) 'Qualitative research: journeys of meaning making through transformation, illumination, shared action and liberation', in Higgs, J., Titchen, A., Horsfall, D. and Armstrong, H. (eds), *Being Critical and Creative in Qualitative Research*, Sydney: Hampden Press, 11–21.

Humphries, B. (2008) *Social Work Research for Social Justice*, Houndmills: Palgrave Macmillan.

Loftus, S., Higgs, J. and Trede, F. (2011) 'Researching living spaces: trends in creative qualitative research', in Higgs, J., Titches, A., Horsfall, D. and Bridges, D. (eds), *Critical Spaces for Qualitative Researching: Living Research*, Rotterdam: Sense, 3–12.

Meinert, R., Pardeck, J. and Kreuger, L. (2000) *Social Work: Seeking Relevancy in the Twenty-first Century*, Binghampton, NY: Hapworth Press.

Morley, C. (2008) 'Developing critical reflection as a research methodology', in Liamputtong, P. and Rumbold, J. (eds), *Knowing Differently: An Introduction to Experiential and Arts-based Research Methods*, New York: Nova Science, 265–80.

——(2009) 'Developing feminist practices', in Allan, J., Pease, B. and Briskman, L. (eds), *Critical Social Work: An Introduction to Theories and Practices*, Crows Nest, NSW: Allen & Unwin, 145–59.

——(2011a) 'Critical reflection as an educational process: a practice example', *Advances in Social Work and Welfare Education: Special Issue – Critical Reflection Method and Practice*, 13(1): 7–28.

——(2011b) 'How does critical reflection develop possibilities for emancipatory change? An example from an empirical research project', *British Journal of Social Work*, 17 November, doi: 10.1093/bjsw/bcr153

Morris, T. (2006) *Social Work Research Methods: Four Alternative Paradigms*, Thousand Oaks, CA: Sage.

Napier, L. and Fook, J. (2000) 'Reflective practice in social work', in Napier, L. and Fook, J. (eds), *Breakthroughs in Practice: Theorising Critical Moments in Social Work*, London: Whiting & Birch, 1–11.

Popkewitz, T. (1984) *Paradigm and Ideology in Educational Research*, New York: Falmer Press.

Powell, J. (2002) 'The changing conditions of social work research', *British Journal of Social Work*, 32: 17–33.

Ramsden, P. (1998) *Learning to Lead in Higher Education*, London: Routledge.

Rossiter, A. (2005) 'Discourse analysis in critical social work: from apology to question', *Critical Social Work*, 6(1): http://www.uwindsor.ca/criticalsocialwork/discourse-analysis-in-critical-social-work-from-apology-to-question

Sands, R.G. (1996) 'The elusiveness of identity in social work practice with women: a postmodern feminist perspective', *Clinical Social Work Journal*, 24(2): 167–86.

Sarantakos, S. (2005) *Social Research* (3rd edn), Houndmills: Macmillan.

Seidman, S. (ed.) (2004) *The Postmodern Turn: New Perspectives on Social Theory*, New York: Cambridge University Press.

Smith, R. (2008) *Social Work and Power*, Houndmills: Palgrave Macmillan.

Taylor, C. and White, S. (2000) *Practising Reflexivity in Health and Welfare: Making Knowledge*, Maidenhead: Open University Press.

White, S. (2001) 'Auto-ethnography as reflexive inquiry: the research act as self-surveillance', in Shaw, I. and Gould, N. (eds), *Qualitative Research in Social Work*, London: Sage, 100–115.

Section 4

Critical reflection in education

15 Critical reflection training to social workers in a large, non-elective university class

Riki Savaya

I first came to critical reflection in 2004, when I was on sabbatical at RMIT University in Melbourne, Australia at a day-long mini-conference organized by Professor Jan Fook and Fiona Gardner at the Centre for Professional Development at La Trobe University. The model presented was based on the use of critical incidents – that is, incidents that are particularly meaningful or significant to the person who experiences them – as objects of reflection. I was moved and impressed by the intense feelings aroused by the process and sensed its potential to help social workers look at underlying meanings and motivations in their practice. I asked Jan and Fiona whether they would be willing to meet with myself and a colleague. They generously offered to undergo the process with us.

Each of us wrote out a critical incident, read it to the others, and reflected on it together. The experience was extraordinarily powerful and meaningful for me. My incident involved my work in evaluating the Couple and Family Counseling Center in Jaffa Tel Aviv, a mixed Jewish Arab area of the city. I found that the Arab population vastly under-used the services in proportion to its numbers in the population despite the well-known prevalence of serious family problems. In order to understand their problems better and to adapt the center's services to their culture and needs, we decided to consult with formal and informal community leaders.

The incident occurred during a meeting I held with a guidance counselor in an Arab high school. At her suggestion, we met at her home, where she lived with her husband and his family. At the door, I was greeted by her mother-in-law, who remained in the living room. In our talk, conducted in Hebrew, the counselor answered my questions about the couple and family problems in the Arab community, how problems are handled traditionally, and the possibilities of integrating the traditional approaches with services offered by the center. After about a quarter of an hour, the counselor's mother-in-law suddenly interrupted the interview in furious tones. Embarrassed, the counselor told me that her mother-in-law thought that she was telling me about her own family problems – in violation of the interdiction in Arab society against telling these to outsiders – and threatened to inform her husband that she had undermined the family's honour. Her efforts to explain to her mother-in-law that our conversation was about problems in the community in general, not their family problems, only enraged her further. I suggested we invite the mother-in-law to join us, but the suggestion came too late, her mother-in-law would not be appeased, and I had to leave.

The incident upset me enormously. The intense sense of failure stayed with me for years, so much so that this incident immediately came to mind in the session with Jan and Fiona more than 10 years later. What bothered me, and what I hoped to clarify by reflecting on the incident, is why it upset me so deeply and for so long. After all, the meeting was with a colleague, in a place of her choosing. Wasn't it her task to make sure that anyone who might be around knew what we were going to discuss before I arrived and that it was alright with them?

The issue wasn't, as it might appear, one of cultural sensitivity. I felt that I had a decent familiarity with and respect for Arab culture, and that our efforts to adapt the center's services to Arab culture and our consultation with Arab leaders were indications of that sensitivity.

The reflection turned out to be extraordinarily illuminating. Through the questions that the others asked and the insights they offered, I came to realize that two central values of mine clashed in this incident: task orientation and inclusion. And I further realized that whenever my task orientation comes into conflict with another value, I invariably choose getting the task done and push aside anything that I see as impeding its efficient completion. Ever since then, I've tried to incorporate this understanding into my practice. I no longer push ahead with the task at hand, come what may. Whenever I find myself pushing aside what I view as an interference to completing a task, I stop to make room for it. From this experience, I also realized how important it is that social workers learn to think critically about their practice and to reflect on the motives and basic assumptions behind their behaviours. As a faculty member in a school of social work, I wrote to the head of the school suggesting an elective course in critical reflection. To my surprise, he made the course mandatory for the entire cohort. I found myself with two classes, one in the fall semester, one in the spring, with forty students each.

In the remainder of this chapter, I describe how I addressed the multiple challenges of bringing critical reflection training using the Fook and Gardner model into a large, mandatory social work class. I use the term 'training' rather than 'teaching' to emphasize that the purpose of the course was to 'train' the students to reflect on their practice, not to 'teach' them about the theories and techniques of critical reflection.

The challenges

Critical reflection can be carried out using a variety of written (journals, jottings, narratives, stories, poems, metaphors, process records) and oral (online discussions, paired or small group processes) forms, or in a combination of the two (Brookfield, 1995; Bolton, 2001; Hunt, 2001; Whipp, 2003; Osmond and

Darlington, 2005). I decided to use the model developed by Fook and Gardner described in chapter 1. In preparing the course, I was confronted with the same challenges and responsibilities faced by all group facilitators using this model: participants' reluctance to reveal their uncertainties, insufficiencies, and mistakes, on the one hand; and their reluctance to probe and challenge other helping professionals about their practice, on the other (Brookfield, 1995; Fook and Askeland, 2007). In addition, I faced the unique challenges of transferring this intimate, voluntary, small group process into a mandatory semester-long course for forty students, in which the facilitator is the same classroom instructor who grades the students' academic performance.

The course

The course was given in the Master of Social Work (MSW) program at the Bob Shapell School of Social Work at Tel Aviv University in Israel. The school's MSW program accepts students who have completed a Bachelor of Social Work, the entry-level degree required for working in the profession in Israel. All of the MSW students are licensed social workers with at least two years of field experience, aged from the mid-twenties through the mid-fifties. Their professional experience and relatively advanced age are advantageous, meaning the students are all likely to have a 'critical incident' from their practice, and have enough professional self-confidence and emotional maturity to benefit from the reflective process. The training focuses on the students' own assumptions and motives, rather than on the incident itself, as is done in other courses.

The model

The course was modeled on the process of critical reflection that I had undergone, which is described in detail in Fook and Gardner's *Practising Critical Reflection* (2007). The model is based on the analysis of a critical incident (Francis, 1997; Fook and Gardner, 2007) using Argyris and Schön's (1974) concept of two theories: espoused theory and theory in-use.

Detailed description

The following account shows how each part of this model was adapted for a class of forty students, in weekly 1.5-hour-long sessions over a 13-week semester.

Introduction (weeks 1–4)

The Introduction occupied the first four classes. Apart from the last class, this was the only part of the course in which all forty students convened together, and the only part in which frontal instruction had a significant place.

The first class meeting opened with a statement concerning the chaotic and highly pressured nature of social work, where practitioners are faced with many uncertainties and crises. This statement was aimed at validating the students' perception of their work as difficult and legitimizing their feelings of frustration and uncertainty, so that they would feel safe to disclose incidents that caused them to feel self-critical, uncomfortable, or upset. The challenge, I told the students, was to identify and examine their spontaneous, unplanned actions, as these reflect their theories-in-use, that is, their basic, often unacknowledged, values, as well as their tacit knowledge. I underscored the point with the Arab proverb 'A camel doesn't see its hump', to which I added, 'unless it's reflected in water'. I explained that the process should make the principles driving their conduct explicit whether the outcome is desirable or not. Up until this point, the role I played was very close to that of the facilitator in more standard critical reflection training workshops.

My first significant divergence was in the presentation of my critical incident. In the original model, the facilitator presents their critical incident along with a written description, and engages in the reflective process with the group members. I distributed a written account of the critical incident from the beginning of this chapter, but without my name, and the students discussed it in groups of four or five persons of their own choosing, for some 20 minutes. I suggested the following general questions: What happened in the incident? What questions would you ask the social worker if she were here? What, in your opinion, could the social worker have done differently? I did not participate in the analyses. Fook and Gardner (2007) emphasize the importance of the facilitator's real-time presentation and reflection as a means of showing him- or herself learning from the process. I could not participate in multiple groups at the same time, and felt that my anonymity was essential to enable the students to speak freely.

Following the groups' separate analyses, a representative of each group presented its observations to the class for discussion. Their responses were used to establish what Fook and Gardner (2007) term a culture or climate of 'critical acceptance', aimed at fostering openness to exposing one's deep assumptions and to learning new perspectives.

The groups' responses tended to be harsh and critical. Some criticized the social worker for lack of cultural sensitivity; a few said she should be fired; others condemned the behaviour of the school counselor. To change the tone, I asked two questions: Do you think that if the social worker or counselor were here, that your responses would foster their desire to reflect on their actions or create resentment, raise their defenses, or paralyze them? How would you feel and respond if you received such responses? These questions brought attention to the judgmental, unsupportive, and unconstructive nature of the students' responses and pointed the way to a more empathic, nuanced, and constructive response style.

I then disclosed that this was an incident of my own, and described the process I underwent, what I had learned about my professional behaviour, and how my learning changed my practice. An instructor's self-disclosure is not common classroom practice. It blurs the hierarchical divide between student and teacher. However, it is essential not only to model the technique of critical reflection, but also to convey first, that it's alright to reveal one's uncertainties and mistakes and second, that we can all learn from our critical reflection to be better practitioners. Instructors fear that self-exposure will erode their authority in the classroom. Just the opposite occurred here. My self-disclosure increased the students' confidence in me as someone who was intimately acquainted with the process I was asking them to undergo and who learned from her critical reflection.

Finally, the students were instructed to write up a critical incident from their own practice and email it to me by the third class. The guidelines were that the critical incident need not be an emergency or crisis, but could be an ordinary, everyday event that they would like to understand better and that was meaningful to them, one they believed they could learn from and felt comfortable sharing with the class. The writing included a brief, focused account of the event itself and the context and background; the students' own behaviours, feelings, and thoughts; and an explanation of why the event was meaningful to them. The accounts ranged between 200 and 1120 words. The analysis of the incidents would begin only in the fifth class. Having the students write them up earlier was aimed at encouraging the beginning of reflection.

The incidents the students brought involved clients, colleagues, and supervisors. Incidents with clients featured clients' hostility and verbal or physical abuse of the social worker, differences between the workers' and clients' perceptions and values, and/or the social worker's difficulties in maintaining boundaries or managing chaotic situations. They raised strong feelings, from fear to frustration and helplessness, undermined the workers' professional self-confidence, and caused them to question their practice, role, and competence. For a fuller account see Savaya et al. (2011). The incidents with colleagues and supervisors involved disagreements about interventions, workers' difficulties in standing up for their professional principles, and lack of support and backup. These incidents raised questions about their ability to represent and advocate for their clients, and feelings of loneliness and isolation.

The second and third classes were devoted to presenting Argyris and Schön's conceptual framework (Argyris, 1974; Argyris and Schön, 1974, 1996).

In the fourth class, students were divided into small groups. The task is a delicate one, as the students will work rather intimately with their group for the entire semester and it is important that they feel comfortable with all the group members. The first time I taught the class, I allocated students to groups based on similarities of themes in their critical incidents. My expectation was that this would best promote joint learning, but some of the groupings were problematic. Students who did not want to work together were forced to do so; students who wanted to work with persons in other groups could not; and students who lived far apart faced logistic difficulties in meeting outside class. Subsequently, the students created their own groupings. Supervisees and supervisors were not placed in the same group, and students' requests not to be in the same group as someone else were respected.

Next, each small group chose one of the four critical incidents written up by its members on which to focus for the remainder of the semester. To facilitate the group selection, I helped the class to establish criteria. First, openness – the student being willing to expose him- or herself and to undergo the critical reflection with others. Secondly, either representativeness or troublesomeness – the incident was representative of other critical events experienced by the members of the group, or involved similar issues, or was particularly troublesome to the student who was psychologically stuck as a result and/or asked to have the group focus on it.

The choice of only one incident for reflection constituted a departure from Fook and Gardner (2007), who maintain that it is essential that every participant present for optimal learning, which also serves to mitigate tendencies towards judgmentalism. Persons who know they will be in the 'hot seat' themselves, they suggest, will be more careful of how they respond to the accounts of others.

This was not feasible for me. Group reflection on a single incident allowed every student to participate in the reflective process. The compromise had the advantage of respecting students who did not want to share their critical incidents with others. Given that the course was mandatory, this provided a way out for the more reserved students.

After each group chose their incident, I divided the class into two groups of twenty students each, such that each half-class group was made up of five small groups. For the rest of the semester, except the last class, each half-class group met in class with me fortnightly, and met without me in their small group in the weeks between. In each half-class session, two critical incidents were analyzed. In the small groups, students continued the analysis. During the deconstruction stage, they modeled the analytical approach of the larger group. During the reconstruction stage, the work started in the small groups and was brought to the larger one. The first half-class began its work in the fifth week of the course, the second half-class in the sixth.

A sample critical incident in the social worker's own words

At 24:00 hours, the night counselor of the hostel [for adolescents in distress] phoned to tell me that one of the boys in my charge was behaving in a strange and unusual way, that he wasn't responding to what he was told to do, that he had a glassy stare, and that his body was shaking. The counselor sounded worried and frightened, and said that he didn't know what to do. Since I was familiar with the boy's emotional background, I decided to go to the hostel, and asked the counselor to notify the hostel's director. When I reached the hostel,

I was informed that the boy had locked himself in the shower room, which increased my worry that he might hurt himself. I asked the counselor to break down the door, which he did. The boy started to scream and to act very violently, which made it difficult to get a hold of him and calm him down. I phoned the hostel director and asked him to come and help us. He apologized and said that he was sick and couldn't come. This reaction made me very angry. I felt alone. And I couldn't believe what I heard. Other night counselors were there and heard the conversation and began to criticize the director very vehemently. I felt exactly like they did, but also that I had to remain loyal to him and not join in the criticism. After a few minutes, the boy lunged towards the window and broke it. He grabbed a shard of glass and began to cut his veins. Seeing the blood, the night counselor went into shock and froze. I was also shocked and I screamed, but I grabbed his hands firmly and, at the same time, asked that a cab be called. While I was holding him, I discovered in myself physical strength that I didn't know I had. The boy is eighteen, about my height, but much stronger than me. Nonetheless, I managed to calm him down. I also discovered emotional strength in myself. Despite my fear and dread and anxiety and anger, and the feeling of being alone, I managed to look composed and confident, which calmed the boy. I spoke to him and told him that we'd be going to the hospital, but he refused adamantly and began to explode again. In the end, I took him to the hospital by myself.

I chose this incident because I feel that it says a lot about my work relations and the way I make intervention decisions. After the incident, I was assailed by a crisis of trust in the system and wanted to quit. I felt that the place did not provide the adolescents or myself with a reliable and professional net of solutions in crisis situations. For several months I went about frustrated and embittered, and almost left for another job. But in the end, the therapeutic relationship I'd built with the adolescents kept me from leaving.

Stage one: Deconstruction (weeks 5–9)

The fifth through ninth weeks are devoted to the deconstruction stage, which aims to help persons examine their fundamental assumptions: the implicit theory-in-use that drives their conduct (Argyris and Schön,1974).

Following Fook and Gardner (2007), the students analyzed the learner's incident using three sets of questions. First, what the presenter's account of the incident implied about his or her fundamental ideals and values, beliefs about power and professionalism, and view of him- or herself and others. It included such questions as: What assumptions, beliefs, attitudes, motivated the presenter's behaviour? What kind of language was used? What stereotypes and prejudices are revealed in the presenter's account? The second set concerned questions about the presenter's understandings of the incident and their behaviours such as: How did the presenter interpret what happened in the incident? How aware was the presenter of the effects of their fundamental assumptions, beliefs, and attitudes on their professional behaviour? What did the presenter expect to happen in the situation? How did those expectations affect the situation? The third set concerned the gaps or contradictions between what the presenter said about what they do and what the incident implies they did. The suggested questions were: What is the gap between what was done and what the presenter intended to do or believed he or she was doing? What questions arise from the description of the incident and your reflections on it about the presenter's behaviour in the incident? The students were given the questions both orally and in writing. They were told that the questions could assist them, but that the questions did not cover everything they might want to ask and that they should raise further questions as they saw fit.

This deconstruction process was presented and modeled in the first half-class meeting, then continued by the students in their small groups. In the half-class meeting, the presenter read her account of the incident; students started with clarifying, then moved on to some of the above probing questions. The presenters were told that they did not have to respond immediately to every question or comment, and could instead take their time, think about the matter, and take it to the small group. This avoided presenters feeling that they were on the spot and provoking a defensive reaction. In the small groups, without exception, the reflective process was taken further and reached considerable depth and intimacy. This point is substantiated in Savaya and Gardner (in press), which discusses the students' reflections on two incidents.

Questions students in the large group asked about the incident

- Why do you feel so angry and frustrated when you functioned so very competently?
- Why did you avoid confronting the director about his behaviour?
- Looking back at the incident, what would you have liked to tell the director? And how would you have said it?
- What do you think the director thought and felt when he was phoned?

Although Fook and Gardner (2007) regard a facilitator as essential to the critical reflection process, the small groups here functioned very well without one. The members worked closely together, knew what questions to ask and how, and had modified the blunt and critical tones they had adopted in the first class. Most demonstrated considerable empathy and were able to offer their insights constructively. They also quickly became self-motivated and self-propelling. Absorbed in a process that they experienced as eye-opening, they invariably met for more than the allotted hour-and-a-half and more than bi-weekly. This, among other things, enabled them to reach the depth of insight they achieved.

Insights about the presenter's motives, values, and behaviours

- Espoused theory regarding work relations.
- Attaining the aims of the work by means of efficient teamwork and the preservation of a pleasant work environment.
- Preserving correct and pleasant relations with persons in authority.
- Properly balancing the client's interests, the needs of the agency, and the worker's personal principles.
- Doing one's job with responsibility, a high work ethic, and serving as a personal example.

Things that kept me from confronting the director

- My fear of my own anger and aggressiveness – that I would lose control of myself if I expressed my anger.
- My fear that the director wouldn't be able to contain my anger and that, in the end, I'd pay a price for it.
- My desire to retain the status and power that I gained by showing that I could handle the difficult incident on my own.
- My deference for authority and tendency to comply.

What I realized about how I communicate

- My way of communicating is unassertive and indirect.
- The reasons are that I fear confrontation and challenging authority, I want to preserve the status quo, and I'm afraid of getting hurt.
- My indirectness and refraining from confrontation had undesirable consequences for the agency. The director didn't know how the staff felt about his inaction and didn't get the chance to explain it. As a result, some of the workers formed a coalition against him and questioned his professionalism and authority.

What I realized about the impression I make

- It's very important for me to project calm, competence, and self-control, even when I'm churning inside.
- People perceive the façade, not the inner upset.
- They see me as a strong and able worker who always manages and doesn't need help.

- The director's refusal to come in the emergency was an expression of his confidence in me.
- My failure to communicate my needs and vulnerabilities causes me a tremendous amount of stress and burnout, and impairs my functioning.

The fact that only one student per group presented their critical incident for reflection was not experienced as limiting. The others reported that they conducted a parallel process on themselves. As the presenter's account was reflected on, they constantly referred to their own critical incidents, asking themselves whether and how the issues raised applied to them, what choices they made in similar situations, what motives really drove their behaviour, and what blind spots they themselves had, and shared their reflections with the group.

Statements by students whose incidents were not the focus of group reflection

- Through the group's reflection on Maya's incident, I identified my own issues with authority, especially masculine authority.
- The reflective process made me think of the issues I encounter with clients in my fieldwork. I realized that it's easier for me to interpret, reflect, and talk about matters that I identify with in my own life. It's harder for me to talk about things I don't see eye-to-eye on because I'm afraid of sounding critical and judgmental.
- I tried to think of my own blind spots, that are inherent in my behaviour. I'm better aware of my own tendency to please my superiors and the great difficulty I have in confronting men in authority ... Maya's reflection made me realize the high price I pay – feelings of loneliness and fear and bearing a heavy load of responsibility on my own – for my need to please and avoidance of confrontation.

By the end of the deconstruction stage, all members of the small groups had gained a new perspective on their professional behaviour, underlying assumptions and values, and disparities between the presenter's espoused theory and theory-in-use.

Stage two: Reconstruction (weeks 10–12)

The students were required to formulate a detailed and well-articulated 'alternative model of practice', including insights from the deconstruction stage, which can also be used by other social workers. The model should serve any of the following.

- Where the aim of the intervention was not attained, it should help the worker to attain it.
- Where the aim was attained, but the worker came away feeling badly about him or herself, it should help to understand and alleviate those negative feelings.
- Where the aims of the intervention were attained and the worker came away feeling empowered, it should present a course of action that other social workers can adopt.

By far the largest number of alternative models were developed to help attain intervention aims that that the students did not attain in their critical incidents.

The reconstruction stage confronted the students with challenges: openness, freedom from defensiveness, readiness to look at one's behaviour and motives with a certain amount of detachment, and the ability to ask questions, cope with uncertainty, and flow with the observations and ideas raised. Most of the MSW students coped well with these tasks.

The challenges posed by the reconstruction process are conceptual, creation of a general abstract alternative model of practice that is clear, detailed, specific, and methodical enough for others to understand its logic and to employ it as a template for action. Many of the students found the conceptual demands difficult.

To help, I established a sequential feedback process. Students composed a rough draft in their small groups. I read these, then met with each small group to clarify and sharpen their formulations and to draw connections between their models and existing models and theoretical frameworks. Students then rewrote their drafts and made a PowerPoint presentation to be presented to the half-class groups. From this, they received further suggestions, which helped them to reformulate their models and achieve greater clarity. The final paper was to be submitted within six weeks after the end of the semester, which is routine in universities in Israel, and has the advantage of allowing time for the students to attain perspective on and consider material in depth.

Summary of the alternative model

The alternative model aims to:

- provide workers with a means of considering the consequences of their decisions for themselves, their agency, and their clients
- avoid the emotional turmoil following upon automatic, impulsive decisions.

Workers must:

- be aware of the hidden motives driving their decisions
- weigh the professional, personal, and ethical costs and benefits of their decisions
- take into account overt and hidden motives in terms of the SWOT model (strengths, weaknesses, opportunities, and threats).

The last class (week 13)

In the last class, in which all forty students were present, I moved to more general observations and questions.

I began by reviewing common themes from the critical incidents, whether or not they had been the focus of group reflection. These included the disparity between the professional value of client empowerment that most of the students espoused and the paternalism that many of them practised; conflicts between personal and professional values; the gap between belief in cooperative collegial relations and competitive feelings and behaviours; questions about the proper exercise of their professional authority; and their problems of self-assertion in the face of opposition or superior authority.

Following the summary, I relayed messages that I felt the students needed to hear, given the bad feelings about themselves that most experienced from their incident, and raised questions for them to think about, including:

- we are not always responsible for others' behaviours
- we cannot control everything our clients or fellow professionals do
- we can't save everyone.

Other messages concerned the alternative models of practice:

- not all the disparities or conflicts that emerged can be resolved.

All these messages must be relayed clearly and firmly, so that the students understand that their inability to solve some dilemmas may stem from the complex realities in which they work, and from the fact that they themselves are a major tool in the intervention process.

I also raised questions that concerned the many disparities and apparent contradictions that emerged, particularly about creating dichotomies, challenging students to consider how polarities are created where reality is more complex.

Second, questions pertaining to clients included:

- How can we deal with situations where our deepest personal values conflict with the values of our clients or of the profession?

- How can we manage situations where we're responsible for helping clients but are not given the resources or backup to do so?
- How can we continue to serve clients who are unappreciative, critical, hostile, or, in some cases, violent?
- How can we use our authority as social workers in a way that respects the rights of others and without undermining or challenging them?
- How can we include the other and give space to all their differences?

The questions pertaining to relations with fellow professionals included:

- How can we work cooperatively with colleagues where there is competition between us?
- How can we make our voices heard, maintain our professional integrity, and stand up for our professional positions when we work in teams where the other members are dismissive or when our status and power are less than theirs?

There was obviously no time to discuss these questions. Nor do they have clear answers. I raised them as a summary of what the critical incidents revealed about the issues with which social workers grapple in their practice, and to leave the students with issues to think about after the course.

The final paper

The final paper consisted of two parts: one written jointly by each small group, one written by each member. In the joint part, they were required to identify the espoused theory, theory-in-use, and the gap between them that emerged in their analysis of the critical incident; to evaluate the effectiveness of the strategies the writer used to attain his or her stated aims; and to present their alternative model of practice. This also meant the group articulated the group process and the product they produced. In the individual paper, each student indicated what he or she learned from the process and whether and how it had affected their practice.

Summary and conclusion

The course has been successful beyond expectations. In their final papers and anonymous feedback forms, the students consistently wrote that it enabled them to learn about their personal and professional selves, compelled them to look inward and attain deeper insights into their practice, and enabled them to identify their blind spots. Many students also stated that critical reflection supplemented the supervision from their workplace. Some wrote that seeing their peers struggle with hidden motives similar to their own tempered the shame and embarrassment they felt and made it easier to face up to and work on these issues. Several wrote that the small group process and course assignments gave structure and a conceptual framework to the reflective process. A fair number of students wrote that this was a model for peer supervision that they would employ in their workplace.

Along with the patent benefits, some problematic issues arose. One was the still too large size of the half-class groups. This was remedied by doubling the number of critical reflection courses given each year, reducing the size of the half-class groups from twenty to ten.

Another issue was the assignment of grades to such a personal and sensitive process. Initially, I tried to tackle the issue by having the students take part in the grade assignment, with small-group members determining 50% of the grade; I determined the other 50% on the basis of the students' final papers. The student-determined grades were inordinately high – between 95 and 100%. After several semesters, I resumed grading the students' work.

A third issue was the uneven quality of the alternative models of practice, sometimes related to student ability, but more often because the problem was not readily remediable (see box). The problem stemmed from the hidden motives that prevented the presenter from confronting her supervisor. But their remedy – that workers identify their hidden motives and weigh them into their decision-making – may be more realistic later than in the pressure of a crisis.

Finally, how can the critical reflection course described in this chapter be adopted by schools of social work in other countries? Its success in Israel depended in some measure on features of the student body, of Israeli culture, and of the university structure. Most of the students were mature individuals, well into their twenties and older, with a fair amount of social work experience. They had the self-confidence that age and experience can bring, and were highly motivated and self-activating. Israeli culture encourages candour and legitimizes risk-taking for men and women. Moreover, the fact that papers can be handed in well after the end of the semester gave the students time to consider the reflection they had conducted from a certain distance and perspective. How well a similar course would succeed with younger, less experienced students, in cultures where openness and direct speech are frowned on, and without the benefit of time to think through the experience before producing a final paper, is an open question.

Based on my own experience of teaching the course, I believe that critical reflection is a powerful tool for improving social work practice. I strongly recommend incorporating a course in critical reflection, with necessary adaptations, as a regular part of social work curricula.

References

Argyris, C.A. (1974) *Behind the Front Page*, San Francisco: Jossey-Bass.
Argyris, C.A. and Schön, D.A. (1974) *Theory in Practice: Increasing Professional Effectiveness*, San Francisco: Jossey-Bass.

——(1996) *Organizational Learning 11: Theory, Method and Practice*, Reading, MA: Addison-Wesley.

Bolton, G. (2001) *Reflective Practice: Writing and Professional Development*, London: Paul Chapman.

Brookfield, S. (1995) *Becoming a Critically Reflective Teacher*, San Francisco: Jossey-Bass.

Fook, J. and Askeland, G.A. (2007) 'Challenges of critical reflection: "Nothing ventured, nothing gained"', *Social Work Education*, 26(5): 520–33.

Fook, J. and Gardner, F. (2007) *Practising Critical Reflection: A Resource Handbook*, Maidenhead: Open University Press.

Francis, D. (1997) 'Critical incident analysis: a strategy for developing critical practice', *Teachers and Teaching: Theory and Practice*, 3: 169–88.

Hunt, C. (2001) 'Shifting shadows: metaphors and maps for facilitating reflective practice', *Reflective Practice*, 3(1): 275–87.

Osmond, J. and Darlington, Y. (2005) 'Reflective analysis: techniques for facilitating reflection', *Australian Social Work*, 58(1): 3–14.

Savaya, R. and Gardner, F. (in press) 'Critical reflection to identify gaps between espoused theory and theory-in-use', *Social Work*.

Savaya, R., Gardner, F. and Stange, D. (2011) 'Stressful encounters with social work clients: a descriptive account based on "critical incidents"', *Social Work*, 56: 63–71.

Whipp, J.L. (2003) 'Scaffolding critical reflection in online discussions: helping prospective teachers think deeply about field experiences in urban schools', *Journal of Teacher Education*, 54(4): 321–33.

16 Critical reflection

Multiple applications within physiotherapy and medicine

Clare Delany and Deborah Watkin

Introduction

In this chapter we describe four different applications of the Fook/Gardner model of critical reflection. These applications incorporate the key features and processes of the model to different degrees. Our applications of the model are examples of using the broad purpose of the model, rather than following the specific procedural steps. Fook and Gardner (2007: 51) describe this broad purpose to 'unsettle the fundamental (and dominant) thinking implicit in professional practice, in order to see other ways of practising'. They also list five more specific purposes of the model which can be used in varying combinations (ibid):

- To develop professional practice theory – by unearthing and then re-developing practice theory.
- To research professional practice – by revealing aspects of practice through a process of articulation and deconstruction in much the same way that research is conducted on practice.
- To evaluate professional practice – by identifying and then comparing implicit assumptions with 'desired thinking and actions'.
- To change professional practice – by identifying and then critically examining dominant assumptions, which can lead to insight for change.
- To learn directly from professional practice experience – by habitually examining and unsettling assumptions about everyday practice.

Three of the applications described in this chapter are in physiotherapy education and one in a workplace orientation program, to assist international medical graduates in making the transition from their overseas experience to the Australian Public Health System. The first application was a six-week critical reflection discussion program for third-year physiotherapy students beginning their first clinical placement. The model of critical reflection for this program followed the small group discussion format, and was informed by the three theoretical components of postmodernism, reflexivity and critical theory (Fook, 2004), as a framework to guide students in their reflection on the nature of professional practice. The second application integrated the same theoretical concepts into the parameters and require-ments of a written critical reflection task about students' clinical placement experiences. The writing task was an individual rather than group discussion-based activity. Students were asked to identify and then analyse a critical incident during their clinical placement using the component theories. The third application was to further embed critical reflection into a series of reflective writing tasks in each semester of the total three-year graduate entry Doctor of Physiotherapy program. The final use of the Fook/Gardner model discussed in this chapter is a structured program of critical reflection for international medical graduates making transitions in the workplace. In this final iteration, we returned to a small-group discussion format to assist new doctors to identify and then compare their past experience with their new working environment.

In this chapter, we demonstrate how each use of the model resulted in a gradual shift along a continuum from using reflection as a separate learning event where we closely followed the Fook/Gardner model including processes and steps of critical reflection, to an embedded learning and teaching process where the components of the reflective model more indirectly informed the teaching and learning task.

Asking students to describe a critical incident in their experience was cen-tral to each of the four critical reflection applications. We found that each use of the model automatically brought us closer to the ideals of adult learning, in particular the theories espoused by Knowles (1970: 45) that adults learn best when they

> Learn how to take responsibility for their own learning through self-directed inquiry, how to learn collaboratively with the help of colleagues rather than compete with them, and, especially, how to learn by analysing one's own experience.

Each successive iteration also demonstrated increasing coherence with Wenger's (1998) notions of legitimate participation. The reflective tasks developed in each of our iterations of the model gradually facilitated students to move from using the component parts of the model to frame how they can learn *from* others to, by the fourth application, being able to learn *with* others. Learners moved from being peripheral participants using structures of reflection, which were somewhat separate from the real learning action, towards a more collaborative learner/teacher structure, where the learners' reflective observations informed the teachers' curriculum development.

We also suggest that successive uses of the model gradually resulted in students more actively incorporating their own experiences into the learning agenda in accordance with the fifth purpose of the model listed above. In this way, critical reflection worked as an enabler of symbiotic curriculum development, that is, curriculum that develops through an active and interdependent relationship between the educator, the organisation deliver-ing the education, and the student. Through the process of critical reflection, students unpacked and critically reviewed their learning experiences and, in so doing, exposed the impact of the curriculum on themselves as the learner. This impact is often hidden from the teacher as the curriculum developer except via formal feedback mechanisms (Nicol and Macfarlane-Dick, 2006). As this effect became obvious, with each application, we set out to inten-tionally exploit this outcome. With each use of the critical reflection model, we were able gradually to dissolve the artificial barrier between learner and teacher. As Fenwick and Tennant (2004: 55) highlight, students are not separate 'objects' from their educator. The position and role adopted by the educator has an impact on how students feel, behave, learn and remember (Fenwick and Tennant, 2004; Delany and Bragge, 2009). Our use of critical reflection demonstrated that students' positioning and understanding of their role and learning experience can and should similarly influence the educator.

Application 1: A critical reflection program for physiotherapy students in their first clinical placement (Delany and Watkin, 2009)

The first critical reflection program closely followed the structured processes of the model outlined by Fook and Gardner (2007). It consisted of a three-hour-per-week small group discussion session scheduled for each week of a six-week clinical placement for third-year physiotherapy students. In this first application, the critical reflection program was separate from students' usual learning events. We drew from the work of (Fook, 2002, 2004) who, writing from a background of social work practice, linked ideas of reflective practice with underlying theoretical bases of postmodernism, reflexivity and critical theory. Fook (2004) used these theories as both definitions and tools of critical reflection to analyse and understand practice or experience. Bleakley (1999) also suggests that highlighting the theoretical background of critical reflection provides a means to interrogate the rigour and relevance of critical reflection as a process in clinical practice. We used these three theore-tical perspectives and the Fook/Gardner model to develop our critical reflection program, where students were guided to deconstruct a learning inci-dent, expose underlying constructs of knowledge, then reconstruct knowledge perspectives and learning strategies.

In the first session, the fourteen participating students were introduced to simplified explanations for the theoretical concepts of postmodernism, critical theory and reflexivity. Students were each asked to identify an event related to their clinical placement to share with the group. They were then guided through stages of reflection by the second author (D.W.) (Delany and Watkin, 2009). These stages included identifying and deconstructing their actions, feelings and different perspectives that were relevant to explaining their incident. From this process, they were then encouraged to develop new ways of constructing knowledge from their experience and ultimately to change their learning work or practice.

Evaluation of the program revealed two key outcomes. First, students reported they had developed enhanced perspectives of their position as learners. Students were able to identify a range of influences on their clinical reasoning, and they described an enhanced awareness of the complexity of health care. Students referred to the impact of power relationships on their learning, and they similarly observed some examples of patients being disempowered within the health care relationships. The students in this first iteration of the model developed an understanding of the hierarchical nature of health care in a large teaching hospital. They reported feeling disenfranchised and lacking an avenue for dialogue within the hospital community (Cranton, 2011), even though uncovering of power relations and social context is often seen as a prelude to enabling social change (Merriam, 2011).

The second key outcome from this program was that critical reflection activities ideally should be embedded within the culture of learning. Students highlighted what they perceived to be the 'one-sidedness' of the critical reflection program. Because critical reflection was not modelled by lecturers or clinical educators, it was seen by students as separate from their other clinical learning. Some students questioned the value of critical reflection, as their immediate supervisory role models, both within the clinical placement and at the university, were not obviously using the reflective processes.

Coherence between the learning environment, professional practice and senior role models is important. As students develop professional identities, the culture of practice displayed by members of the profession is highly influential to learning with, joining and belonging to a professional community (Knowles et al., 2005). Fish (2005) suggests developing a professional identity is the first stage of professionalisation, which is followed by critically appraising professional frameworks and continually redefining what it is to be that professional.

The outcomes of this first iteration demonstrate that, whilst the program did achieve a common language to discuss, identify and include the sociocultural, heuristic and ethical components of clinical practice, it was ultimately separate from what students perceived as the real learning agenda (Delany and Bragge, 2009). Students reported that, although useful to their own professional development, the program was not sufficiently embedded in their work or the professional culture they were joining, lacking role modelling by significant others. Based on this review, three factors were identified as potential limits to the absorption or integration of critical reflection into the fabric of health professional practice (Delany and Molloy, 2009):

- a focus on description and analysis of incidents and practice rather than a prompt to use the reflection to change and challenge practice
- a lack of vertical integration of reflective tasks in the academic program for incremental building of critical reflection skills
- a lack of modelling of critical reflection by both academic and clinical staff.

Application 2: Critical reflection in clinical education: beyond the swampy lowlands (Delany and Molloy, 2009)

In our second application of the Fook/Gardner model, we addressed the learning outcomes and lessons of the first iteration, specifically to integrate the process of reflection with the experience of learning and practice. In the second application, the goal was to draw from the overall purposes of the Fook/Gardner model by encouraging students to recognise obvious and less obvious assumptions underpinning their experiences of learning on clinical placement, and to guide them to move purposefully between theories explaining their experiences. We called this approach an 'iterative model of critical reflection'. Based on qualitative research paradigms (Hansen, 2006), the key goals of this model were to encourage students to engage in critical reflection by moving dynamically between underpinning theories to inform and explain practice, in much the same way that they rely on theories of practice to inform their clinical discipline-based knowledge. We diverged from the Fook/Gardner model by focusing on students' individual reflective activity rather than using the socially mediated learning that comes from the small group reflection. This was a pragmatic divergence based on the need to provide a cohort of sixty students with 'an experience' of using critical reflection.

In this second application we could not rely on a facilitator modelling the process of reflective questioning. We therefore set out first to provide second-year physiotherapy students on their first clinical placement with more explanation, via formal lectures, of the underpinning theories about critical reflection, to enhance their ability to access concepts and language. The second aim was to set an independent assignment where students were encouraged to move beyond 'description' into critical analysis; and the third, to guide students to generate strategies for improved learning and practice. The fourth aim was explicitly to incorporate students' reflections back into the developing curriculum. The broad purposes of critical reflection, stated in the Fook/Gardner model – to research and change professional practice – underpinned our goals for this activity. However, because of the context of undergraduate learning, we offered this opportunity in the form of a structured assignment with outcomes of feeding back the general outcomes of reflection back into the curriculum.

Drawing from the work of Johns (1995), we used three marking criteria to encourage this more critical and dynamic connection with the curriculum, through to students' reflective writing. Students' essays were formally evaluated for their capacity to challenge assumptions through structured reflection; for their level of critical discussion of relevant cultural, ethical and professional issues; and for their ability to demonstrate analysis of potential discrimination within the situation. The following questions guided students to achieve these reflective writing goals:

• How does the writing demonstrate linking of theory to practice appropriate to the students' area of learning?

- How does the writing demonstrate the use of resources and their application?
- What level of critical reflection, using analysis, synthesis and evaluation, does the writing demonstrate?

Chur-Hansen (2008) suggests that one of the most valuable teaching and learning outcomes from ongoing examination of students' portfolio writing was the ability of the educator to understand better how and why student learning difficulties arise, as they arise. With this in mind, students' written observations, analysis and reflection were collected and then translated into pragmatic curricula or institutional changes. For example, the topic of death and dying was raised by many students. This topic was subsequently introduced into the curriculum in their following undergraduate year, through the introduction of a lecture and a case-based learning scenario centred on palliative care. The theme of negotiating relationships, raised by students in many of their essays, was addressed through the inclusion of a 'non-technical skills' session in the pre-clinical transition week, involving students practising skills of negotiation with simulated or standardised patients.

This form of modelling, where learners can see the links between inquiry, critical thinking and change, is essential in helping shape students' construction of reflection as part of practice, rather than a metacognitive add-on to their learning in clinical practice (Delany and Molloy, 2009). It is also a key underpinning purpose of the Fook/Gardner model. Moving iteratively between student insight, knowledge and evaluation, and development of educational content and teaching methods reflects our underpinning theoretical stance on reflective practice. That is, that reflective practice is not just about 'contemplation and analysis', but also about transformative change.

In a business setting, Robbins et al. (2009) point to a continually evolving environment where organisations need constantly to learn, adapt and change. This is also pertinent to the health care environment, where the insights and learning of students enable the teacher and the teaching organisation to respond by reviewing teaching practice and adjusting and developing clinical practice strategies to suit the clinical environment as experienced by students. This acquired knowledge about current health care practice can then be incorporated as teaching transformation (Knowles et al., 2005). This process underscores the potential value of critical reflection as a valuable process to unpack complex knowledge and identify practical actions (Dubrin et al., 2006).

Application 3: Critical Perspectives in Physiotherapy Program within the Doctor of Physiotherapy Program, The University of Melbourne

The graduate entry physiotherapy doctoral program began its first year in 2011 at the University of Melbourne. In developing this curriculum, there was a need to ensure the capabilities of students who had already completed one degree were acknowledged and built upon. A key principle of adult learning, identified by Knowles et al. (2005), is to assist students to be involved in formulating the curriculum or, in Wenger's (1998) terms, to move a student from the periphery towards the centre of a community of learning. The shift to a professional doctorate degree provided an opportunity to revise critical reflection subjects to integrate with each other, and to utilise learning and teaching methodologies that are more 'postgraduate in nature'.

More postgraduate in nature can be understood, typically, as students having a more active role in their own learning, and becoming creators of knowledge and innovation rather than consumers of knowledge. From this basis, the subject 'Critical Perspectives in Physiotherapy' was developed. The tasks are embedded within one subject for each semester of the course, comprising 15% of the total mark in each subject. The series of critical reflective tasks were designed to build incrementally students' capacity to critically reflect on their own thinking and learning, and their interactions with supervisors and patients. Each critical reflection task represents a building block in the development of critical reflection skills. The overriding goals are to foster an awareness of the language, professional discourse and practice philosophy, and make these concepts accessible to students. More specifically, each task aimed to 'unsettle' students' 'assumptions about practice' (Fook and Gardner, 2007: 51).

Due to the large (eighty-student) cohort, we focused on the main principles of the model rather than using small groups, with time built in for individual participation. We developed marking criteria to direct students to identify and deconstruct fundamental aspects of physiotherapy learning and practice and underpinning assumptions. We also encouraged students to identify alternative approaches and theories relevant to physiotherapy education and clinical practice.

The first Critical Perspectives in Physiotherapy assignment required students to reflect on how physiotherapy skills were taught and how they, as learners, engaged with them. The second assignment challenged students to recognise that physiotherapy practice, although grounded in technical skills and evidence-based knowledge, draws both implicitly and explicitly from philosophical, ethical and technical interests, theories and paradigms. These include (Trede and Higgs, 2009):

- health care ethics, philosophy and values
- positivist/empiricist research and knowledge
- social/constructivist views of knowledge and reality
- theories of sociology and humanity
- physiotherapy-specific values
- physiotherapy-specific technical interests
- critical perspectives.

The second assignment asked students to explore two of these theories by applying them as an explanatory framework to a critical incident in their first clinical placement. Years 2 and 3 in this program are planned for 2012 and 2013. The critical reflection assignments designed for year 2 (2012) and year 3 (2013) will build on the first two assignments by requiring students to move from reflecting on sources of knowledge informing physiotherapy practice education (semester 1); through theoretical explanations of physiotherapy practice (semester 2); to a phenomenological analysis of a patient's experience of illness (via qualitative in-depth interview) (semester 3); using art and literature as an explanatory frame for health and illness (semester 4); a reflection on ethics, professionalism and leadership (semester 5); and an opportunity to develop their own philosophy of practice within the physiotherapy profession as the final-semester reflective task (semester 6).

The tasks are designed developmentally because they gradually build up students' capacity to develop their own understanding of physiotherapy professional practice theory; skills to research their own professional practice and learning; and strategies to both deconstruct and reconstruct their professional practice behaviours. Each reflective task is designed to facilitate students to be reflexive about their positions as physiotherapists, to recognise a range of different perspectives, and to adopt a critical gaze about their approach and their patients' experiences. The third application also embeds the process of critical reflection into the fabric of learning throughout a physiotherapy program.

Application 4: Transition in practice – a critical reflection group for new doctors

This program of critical reflection used an informal setting (a lunchtime discussion session) to facilitate interactions between new doctors making the transition from overseas experience to an Australian Public Health System. In this final iteration, we returned to the processes of the Fook/Gardner model. The group was conducted with a facilitator and each person was encouraged to talk about their experiences in practising medicine from their specific cultural background. Our specific purpose was to encourage participants to research their professional practice by deconstructing their own ideas about a particular clinical area of practice and compare that interpretation with the practice as described by a local hospital staff member. We also drew directly from concepts of situated learning within a community of practitioners in the workplace (Lave and Wenger, 1991), because the program sought to move beyond considering senior medical professionals as the only teachers of new doctors. We invited a diverse range of hospital staff to the discussion group, including radiographers, bed coordinators, medical records staff and porters, all of whom were integral to new doctors' orientation to their local system. The critical reflection process followed a simple structure and series of questions. The new doctors began the discussion and were asked to respond to the following questions about a particular area of their practice:

- What are some of the issues/challenges you experience when working with … (a social worker; physiotherapist; medical records department radiographer)?
- What are some of the most important aspects of working in this area?
- What was your previous experience of working in this area?
- What expectations do you have of this area of practice?

Following their description of their experiences and particular challenges, they then listened to a guest speaker (an old-timer) from within the hospital. The guest speaker presented their expertise and practice; how they fitted into the health system; and tips and strategies for accessing and using their service for new doctors. They were asked to respond to the following types of question:

- Could you tell us what a typical day looks like?
- What expectations do you have of the doctors?
- What do you think makes a good referral to your service?
- What are some common challenges faced by new doctors in accessing your service?

The key aspects of this critical reflection program were to:

- consider new doctors as educators as well as learners – the program was designed to provide space for doctors to teach themselves about the system within which they were working, in a supportive setting
- focus on new doctors sharing their experiences and reflections on their observations – the program was interactive and supported doctors to talk about and make sense of their own experiences
- provide, through a structured reflection model, a method of learning and problem-solving in clinical practice.

This program of critical reflection explicitly acknowledged the challenges experienced by skilled practitioners transitioning to new environs, and sought to assist them to explore those challenges and identify areas of learning need. The program was designed for doctors to *teach themselves* about the system as they are working within it, in a supportive setting, through sharing experiences and reflections on their observations, methods of learning and problem-solving in clinical practice. A further unique aspect of this program was that it facilitated interactions between new doctors, mostly international medical practitioners and other local staff members, all of whom are integral to new doctors' orientation to their local system. Wenger (1998: 100) writes that 'it is only through spending time with old-timers that [newcomers] can become part of the community. Old-timers introduce the newcomers into the actual practice of the community.' This is a de-centred approach that is about learning in the 'community of practice' rather than from a master (Lave and Wenger, 1991: 94).We also aimed to develop what Fook and

Gardner (2007: 78) refer to as 'a culture of critical acceptance', where the new doctors felt supported, safe and respected enough to encourage learning and professional growth.

Based on weekly feedback collected at the completion of each session, the program succeeded on a number of levels. Firstly, it provided a forum for new doctors to critically reflect upon their observations of differences in practice, between their past and present work environments. As adjustment entails a constant oscillation between the past and present clinical work, it is important to have space in which to reflect on the importance and implications of difference. For some doctors, differences were striking, such as not previously encountering particular staff members such as social workers and pharmacists. For other doctors, it was an awareness that the system was different from what they were used to. The critical reflection program was emancipatory in that it provided them with tools to negotiate a system that was complicated and confusing. The program also focused upon everyday practices, such as writing drug charts, making a physiotherapy referral and filling in discharge summaries. Invited staff members brought forms with them to the meeting, which contributed a level of materiality to these discussions.

According to their feedback about the program, new doctors developed insights into the local system and better awareness of the roles of staff members, while visiting staff learnt more about new doctors' expertise and past experiences. Program participants indicated that they had more confidence to ask questions in the workplace of various staff members, who were seen as 'friendly, helpful and capable', and had developed a range of practical strategies helpful for their everyday tasks. The doctors found the program encouraging and supportive of their situation.

This final application of both the broad goals and the structure of the Fook/Gardner model represents a form of action learning as a group, where collaborative inquiry via repeated episodes of reflection and action occurs within a group (Cranton, 2011). A common process of learning and orientation for new doctors involves listening (passively) to a senior doctor, who passes on relevant information. This process means the learner and educator are not equal. We set out, through a process of reflection and dialogue in the workplace, to bring greater coherence and equality between learner and teacher (Mayo, 2011).

Conclusion

This chapter highlights four applications of the Fook/Gardner model. From an overall perspective, the different uses demonstrate two key phenomena. The first is a gradual absorption into the learning task of the formal theories of postmodernism, reflexivity and critical theory. This phenomenon of formal frameworks and theories of practice becoming less visible with increasing familiarity and use is apparent in literature examining the practice of experts in a range of fields. Experts' thinking and sources of knowledge and experience convert to a type of tacit knowledge where they seem to just know what to do or how to frame and solve a problem (Higgs, 2008). As our familiarity with the theories underpinning, and overall purposes of, critical reflection grew, our ability to flexibly merge and embed the theories throughout a full curriculum (see the third iteration within the Doctor of Physiotherapy program) and within the fabric of everyday clinical practice (see the fourth iteration for international medical graduates) suggests a shift towards more expert use of the overriding purposes articulated in the model. The second explanatory phenomenon to emerge from our changing use of the model is that the model itself is inherently robust and flexible, and therefore capable of adjusting to a range of different applications (Thomas, 1997).

Our description of four different applications of the Fook/Gardner model highlights a process of reflection as curriculum designers. We began with a structured application of the model. We gradually merged the model, and in particular its key purposes, into the process and fabric of a range of student learning experiences. Our flexible use of the model resulted in learners taking increasing responsibility for their own reflection about practice, with such reflection becoming an intrinsic component of their everyday decision making.

References

Bleakley, A. (1999) 'From reflective practice to holistic reflexivity', *Studies in Higher Education*, 24: 315–30.

Chur-Hansen, A. (2008) 'Keeping a journal of reflections on learning', in Facione, N.C. and Facione, P.A. (eds), *Critical Thinking and Clinical Reasoning in the Health Sciences: An International Multidisciplinary Teaching Anthology*, Millbrae, CA: California Academic Press.

Cranton, P. (2011) 'Adult learning and instruction: transformative learning perspective', in Rubenson, K. (ed.), *Adult Learning and Education*, Oxford: Elsevier/Academic Press.

Delany, C. and Bragge, P. (2009) 'A study of physiotherapy students' and clinical educators' perceptions of learning and teaching', *Medical Teacher*, 31: 402–11.

Delany, C. and Molloy, E. (2009) 'Critical reflection in clinical education: beyond the "swampy lowlands"', in Delany, C. and Molloy, E.K. (eds), *Clinical Education in the Health Professions*, Sydney: Elsevier.

Delany, C. and Watkin, D. (2009) 'A study of critical reflection in health professional education: "Learning where others are coming from"', *Advances in Health Sciences Education*, 14: 411–29.

Dubrin, A., Miller, P. and Dalglish, C. (2006) *Leadership*, Milton: Wiley Press.

Fenwick, T. and Tennant, M. (2004) *Understanding Adult Learners*, Crows Nest: Allen & Unwin.

Fish, D. (2005) 'The anatomy of educational evaluation in clinical education, mentoring and professional supervision', in Rose, M. and Best, D. (eds), *Transforming Practice through Clinical Education: Professional Supervision and Mentoring*, London: Elsevier.

Fook, J. (2002) 'Theorizing from practice: towards an inclusive approach for social work research', *Qualitative Social Work*, 1: 79–95.

——(2004) 'Critical reflection and transformative possibilities', in Davies, L. and Leonard, P. (eds), *Social Work in a Corporate Era: Practices of Power and Resistance*, London: Ashgate.

Fook, J. and Gardner, F. (2007) *Practising Critical Reflection: A Resource Handbook*, Maidenhead: Open University Press.

Hansen, E. (2006) *Successful Qualitative Health Research*, Sydney: Allen & Unwin.

Higgs, J. (2008) *Clinical Reasoning in the Health Professions*, Edinburgh: Butterworth-Heinemann.

Johns, C. (1995) 'Framing learning through reflection within Carper's fundamental ways of knowing in nursing', *Journal of Advanced Nursing*, 22: 226–34.

Knowles, M. (1970) *The Modern Practice of Adult Education: Andragogy versus Pedagogy*, New York: Association Press.

Knowles, M.S., Holton, E.F. and Swanson, R.A. (2005) *The Adult Learner*, London: Elsevier.

Lave, J. and Wenger, E. (1991) *Situated Learning: Legitimate Peripheral Participation*, Cambridge: Cambridge University Press.

Mayo, P. (2011) 'Adult learning, instruction and program planning: insights from Freire', in Rubenson, K. (ed.), *Adult Learning and Education*, Oxford: Elsevier.

Merriam, S. (2011) 'Adult learning', in Rubenson, K. (ed.), *Adult Learning*, Oxford: Elsevier.

Nicol, D. and Macfarlane-Dick, D. (2006) 'Formative assessment and self-regulated learning: a model and seven principles of good feedback practice', *Studies in Higher Education*, 31: 199–218.

Robbins, S., Bergman, R., Stagg, I. and Coulter, M. (2009) 'Management yesterday and today', in Robbins, S., Bergman, R., Stagg, I. and Coulter, M. (eds), *Foundations of Management*, Frenchs Forest, NSW: Pearson Education.

Thomas, G. (1997) 'What's the use of theory?', *Harvard Educational Review*, 67: 75–103.

Trede, F. and Higgs, J. (2009) 'Models and philosophy of practice', in Higgs, J., Smith, M., Webb, G., Skinner, M. and Croker, A. (eds), *Contexts of Physiotherapy Practice*, Sydney: Churchill Livingstone.

Wenger, E. (1998) *Communities of Practice: Learning, Meaning, and Identity*, Cambridge: Cambridge University Press.

17 Critical reflection in social work education

Roslyn Giles and Rosalie Pockett

Students' relationship with values and knowledge

Working with, and accepting, diversity and difference are key elements in social work practice. Finding effective ways to facilitate and support students' understandings of these concepts in a complex world provides many challenges for social work education. To meet these challenges, the integration of critical reflection into the developmental stages of student learning has been one of the cornerstones of the social work curriculum at the University of Sydney. Elements of Fook's critical deconstruction and reconstruction approach (Fook, 2002) and the Fook and Gardner model (2007) have been adapted and integrated into a prolonged engagement with students in their final two years of the degree.

The overall programme is grounded in a commitment to the provision of high-quality social work education that fosters critical and informed engagement with theory, policy and practice; the promotion of a strong relationship between research, scholarship and teaching; and building partnerships with academic, policy and practitioner partners. Central to these commitments is the understanding that social work is about a commitment to tackling social injustices and inequalities through political and social engagement with the issues of the day. In addressing these principles, the programme aims to prepare graduates for employment in an environment that is complex, diverse and changing, and where capacity to transfer knowledge and skills across contexts is essential. To this end, the programme engages with key strategies to build on prior learning, to demand greater responsibility for learning, and to motivate students towards a commitment to lifelong learning. Graduating students are expected to be reflexive, versatile and skilful in diverse contexts of practice, and to be able to translate professional values into action. Along with field education, the curriculum includes issue-based learning approaches that connect policy, research, professional skills and fields of practice (Irwin and Napier, 2004). Central to this learning is the ability to understand and act on the concept and processes of critical thinking.

Throughout this chapter, we use a number of terms in discussing social work education that are nuanced in meaning. For our purposes, critical thinking is the process where a student moves beyond description to a deeper, analytical and evaluative approach. Reflexivity is an active process of critically analysing the knowledge and values that influence practice. Taylor and White (2000) suggest this is 'epistemic reflexivity', which is achieved when social workers *and students* (sic) become aware of the dominant discourses and the tacit assumptions (Polanyi, 1967) that underpin their practice. In using the term critical reflection, we are using the approach developed by Fook and Gardner (2007) that is 'a process (and theory) for unearthing individually held social assumptions in order to make changes in the social world' (p. 14). Thus the interrelationships between context, theory and practice, and social change are key elements. Combining these approaches into a learning experience that supports integration, synthesis and growth is referred to as transformational learning.

Pedagogical overview

Critical reflection sits comfortably within social work education for both epistemological and pedagogical reasons. Epistemologically, there is a synergy with contemporary educational theories that aim for transformative and deep learning based on the integration and convergence of knowledge and experience into practice. The early work of higher education theorists such as Biggs (1978, 1996) and Prosser et al. (1994) conceptualised student learning in an interactive model known as the 'presage, process and product model' of student learning. Using this model as an example, the challenge for social work educators is to incorporate critical reflection into the 'process' stage of learning whilst drawing on the life experiences and expectations that students bring to the course, that is, 'presage'. This needs to be undertaken in a way that achieves students' proficiency in all the elements that underpin practice, including theoretical frameworks and approaches, values and ethical stances, skill development, and the contextual bases of practice. Collectively, these would be referred to in the model as the 'product' or the achievement of learning outcomes. In doing so, educators would aim for the constructive alignment (Biggs, 1996) or internal coherence of learning, experience and meaning-making. Contemporary theorists have identified the need in student education to build understanding and engagement with learning for the twenty-first century as a priority for university education (McCune and Entwistle, 2011). Learning environments that support students' 'will to learn' (Barnett, 2007), and the more recent iteration of 'a disposition to understand for oneself' (McCune and Entwistle, 2011), build on concepts such as Biggs' constructive alignment to prepare students for what Barnett calls the 'supercomplexity' of the contemporary world and the personal demands of working in a 'climate of uncertainty' facing 'more and more unanswerable questions' (p. 303).

Transformational learning for transformational practice

Achieving socially just, effective practice in a 'climate of uncertainty' and supercomplexity is supported by engaging with concepts of transformational learning that lead to and underpin transformational practice.

> By transformational learning we mean significant learning experiences that engage the learner intellectually, emotionally and socially. Transformational learning moves the learner beyond the attainment of factual knowledge into his/her own experience, thinking and meaning making. The learner has opportunities to reflect on and analyse their learning, build onto their previous learning, and assess the relevance of this learning for a future situation.
>
> (Giles et al., 2010: 7)

Central to transformational learning is the ability to move from reflection to critical reflection and critically reflective practice. Such practice 'emphasizes the power of agency, both personal and collective, to transform society' (Agger, 1998: 5). Understanding and acting on power is essential in the process of surviving and thriving in human services and the political context of organisations. Without this practitioners can become left-behind, bitter, self-defeating and powerless. Understanding the subtleties of power can mean the difference between staying in an organisation and leaving; between creating change within social systems and accepting unjust and inhumane practices; between engendering inner empowerment and self-efficacy and remaining apathetic. Ensuring that critical reflection becomes a natural and routine part of future practice underpins the deep learning approaches within the programme (Clare, 2007; Giles et al., 2010). It also supports the contention by Brookfield (2009) that one of the key benefits of critical reflection is enabling practitioners *and students* (sic) to 'keep a sense of perspective on the limits of their influence' (p. 294).

Adaptation of the model in social work curricula

Critical reflection presents some intrinsic challenges for social work educators who are both enabling students to build sound foundations for practice and, at the same time, challenging many conceptual aspects of these same foundations. 'Shaking up assumptions' can be challenging for students. The reassurance of 'certainty' has been identified as a key driver for students (Taylor and White, 2006). Similarly, demands from external stakeholders in the profession such as accrediting bodies (AASW, 2010), employers and practitioners seek assurance that social work curricula contain a foundational knowledge base for professional practice.

The use of specific tools, in particular the critical incident technique (Fook, 2002) and elements of the Fook and Gardner model (2007), which emphasise the incorporation of new understandings into the 'theory to practice' relationship, have supported the successful integration of this approach into the curriculum, and help to address the potential binaries that may arise between critical thinking, technical proficiency and professional practice. These approaches enable the exploration and analysis of situations and experiences that build meaning for the individual student and also provide a means by which reworked narratives and ways of understanding aid the formulation of new theories and approaches to practice within commonly agreed principles and values. They can be used with individuals as well as small groups, thus making them adaptable and responsive to student education.

The concepts of critical reflection and reflexivity are introduced to students through the specific design of assessment activities through the course. These assessments progressively support students' abilities to think critically about their work, in addition to mastering the theory and practice requirements of a professional degree.

Social work educators as facilitators

In the final two years of the undergraduate degree, all student assessments include marking criteria that assess students' abilities in critical analysis and reflection. In doing so, social work educators act in a similar role to that of the facilitator/s in the Fook and Gardner model, in particular, 'the broader role … in establishing and maintaining the critical reflection culture' based on a commitment to the process and an ability to model the process through the course. Feedback is often given to students by posing a number of questions that have the effect of 'unsettling the assumptions' that may be evident in the piece of work. Thus, consistent with the aims of the first stage of the model, the feedback from teachers aims 'to help each student articulate some changed and meaningful awareness of their experience' (Fook and Gardner, 2007: 73).

Within the professional practice units of study, staged skill development is undertaken using educational approaches, case studies and texts that use a critically reflective approach (O'Hara and Pockett, 2011). These pre-field education courses aim to develop knowledge, skills and values central to effective interpersonal actions. Taking a developmental and staged approach each week, students participate in experiential exercises where actions and reflections on these actions promote understanding and skills in respectful, genuine, non-oppressive practice. An example of a beginning exercise requires students to explore their personal values. In this exercise, students are asked to consider their response to statements specifically developed around selected current social issues, for example:

- 'Smacking children should be against the law.'
- 'Children should be removed from families where violence towards them is continuous.'
- 'Alcohol should be legally available to those under eighteen years of age.'

Students in the class form a line across the classroom, locating their position on the continuum ranging from definitely 'yes' to definitely 'no', and then debate their positions. Students discuss what informs these values, how their individual understandings support or clash with assumed and dominant values, and the impact this may have on their future practice. In reflection about the exercise, students consistently find their worldview challenged and altered when other positions are articulated and 'unpacked'.

Another exercise involves students role-playing particular case scenarios, taking on the roles of all the participants, as in the following example.

> You are working as a social worker in a hospital maternity ward and you have received a referral from the nursing staff to visit a young Koori woman, Corenna (fifteen years old), who has just given birth to a baby girl. Nursing staff referred Corenna to you because of concerns about her wellbeing and that of her newborn child. Corenna presented at the hospital only hours before giving birth, and it seems she has not accessed prenatal services during the course of her pregnancy. The baby is substantially underweight, and will need to gain weight before being released from hospital. Nursing staff are concerned that Corenna may be drug-dependent and this may have contributed to the baby's low birth weight. Corenna's mother, grandmother and older sister were present at the birth and appear very supportive of her. As far as the nursing staff have been able to ascertain, Corenna is no longer with the father of the child, and she plans to live with her mother and sister in their two-bedroom high-rise apartment on leaving hospital.
>
> (Case scenario developed by class teachers,
> based on practice experience)

Through taking on different roles in the scenario, students experience first-hand how differing values, beliefs and knowledge affect human service delivery. In the early class work, students usually want to focus on how to solve the presenting problem in the case study. Their experiential learning is guided by class teachers acting as facilitators. In later classes, case scenarios are often revisited, and students are asked to rewrite the scenarios being mind-ful of the theoretical lens through which they are presenting the information, and the assumptions, values and discourses that inform and influence this process. In each of these exercises, students also begin to understand the concept of a 'critical friend' – engaging in a dialogue with another person that assists with the analysis of the kinds of thinking and constructions that influenced their account of an experience (Fook, 2002: 99).

Supporting and nurturing students' readiness and ability to open themselves up to this type of learning is a key role of social work educators; and in particular, ensuring this learning is continued in field education. Field educa-tion includes two extended periods of field-based practice learning. Learning agreements are developed for each student that incorporate all the elements of professional social work practice underpinned by critical reflection approaches (Giles et al., 2010). The success of this approach is dependent on educators' skill in guiding students and students' receptiveness to the process. Each field educator is provided with material about the concept and process of critical reflection. In addition to agency-based field education, students also participate in campus classes where they consider issues such as the context of practice, including organisational culture and theoretical approaches. In peer-support groups designed to develop their 'critical friend' skills, students are asked to reflect on placement experiences such as statutory and other work with involuntary clients, and ethical dilemmas in practice. These reflections are then presented to the larger class in a manner that promotes further debate and knowledge development.

Student feedback regarding the impact of these combined educational experiences is reflected in their comments about significant learning at the conclusion of field education:

> linking theory to practice is key to learning in field education (student A)
> good supervision is essential to attaining skills in critical reflection in practice (student B)
> challenging my own personal worldviews – seeing differences, what is informing and how valid are my assumptions (student C)
> significant for me was understanding and working with tensions in the workplace – personal/professional values; organisational values and then considering the concept of advocacy ... the 'when and how' (student D).

Formulating the narrative and power discourses

Two key areas that challenge student learning in the use of critical reflection are first, the ability to step outside the narrative or 'stay outside the story' (Fook and Gardner, 2007: 82) that they have developed about a situation or issue; and second, their understandings about relationships of power within the narrative that they have constructed to understand their experience. It is usually the case that students' early constructions of power are based on their own experiences of powerlessness rather than powerfulness. This is exemplified in the first assignment, which specifically incorporates a critical reflective stance.

Students are asked to write an individual critical reflection about their experiences in a team project that they have just completed. In this project, students are randomly divided into small teams to complete a social work-related activity, for which the team receives a mark. The aim of the experiential team activity is to introduce students to working interprofessionally. The theories that inform the tasks are related to small group theories (Douglas, 2000; O'Hara, 2011) and interprofessional practice (Payne, 1982; Craddock et al., 2006; Payler et al., 2007). The collaborative process is not always a smooth one, and the team mark, which is also an individual mark, may not reflect students' individual academic performance: some students who would normally be in a pass grade range for individual work may receive a very high mark for this piece of work if their team mark was high; conversely, students who would normally receive distinctions and high distinctions individually may receive a much lower mark if their team mark was low.

The team experience for each student acts in a similar way to a 'critical incident', particularly if the team encountered difficulties. Students are asked to critically reflect on what happened in their team, their role, and what they learned from the experience.

Stepping out of the experience is a challenging task for most students. At this early stage of understanding, students' comments and analysis still remain self-centric, demonstrating the difficulty of developing a narrative in which they can remain 'outside the story'. This is probably the most difficult part of student learning, as students are being asked to be self-aware and to develop understandings and interpersonal skills that support their identity as social workers; and at the same time, by using critical reflection, are being asked to step outside this frame. This is compounded further for students who have not yet been on placement and who lack grounding in a social work practice environment.

Some examples of assumptions that are not clearly articulated by students at this stage are that teamwork is an effective way to work together with other professionals. A taken-for-granted assumption is made about this, based on the content of material presented in lectures and readings. The way teams have been formed is also a taken-for-granted assumption – a random allocation of students based on their tutorial groups will provide a work-like context in which experiential learning will take place. Two further assumptions are identified by some students in their reflections: the assumption that their teams will work because they are *social work* students, which somehow imbues them with all the understandings and insight necessary to work effectively with others; and the assumption that there is no need for a team leader in teams of social work students, as these taken-for-granted qualities will enable a democratic, conciliatory and consensus-building approach to problem-solving.

Some examples of students' experiences, documented in their critical reflection, include the following.

> From the initial meeting of our group, I felt like an outsider as many members of our group were also friends ... they bonded into a kind of sub-group ... this created a dynamic that was never addressed in the group. (student 1)
>
> Upon reflection, I should have taken my issues to the group, instead of letting my feelings build up. (student 2)

My approach to critical reflection consisted of writing a narrative of my experience of working interprofessionally ... one individual within the group did not contribute in the planning or presentation of the project ... I held the assumption that team members should participate equally but this did not occur in our team. (student 3)

I have blamed the group for the unequal distribution of work. However, I have had similar experiences in other groups. When I reflect on my own role in the group, I can see that my enthusiastic personality has meant that I end up doing more work than other group members. (student 4)

This exercise also tests their assumptions about friendship and peer-group relationships. The majority of small teams usually do not nominate a team or group leader, and this is justified using terms such as 'collaboration', 'partnership', 'consensus' and 'equality'. Some students make excellent attempts to analyse their team's processes using small group theories and those of interprofessional practice; however, the critical examination of their own experiences and the as-yet-unstated and -unspoken binary positions set up at the outset are not well articulated. At this early stage, students are able to identify some of the assumptions they made about their student colleagues and analyse these against their own experiences and beliefs about how teams should work together.

To demonstrate the staged development of understanding and ability to undertake this process, comments from final assignments can be compared. A 'capstone' assignment is set for students who have fully completed their field education and have returned to the university to undertake a final integrative unit of study. This assignment provides a means through which many students demonstrate transformational learning. The assignment, developed by our academic colleague Deb Hart, involves students submitting a manuscript for publication in response to a call for papers for a special 'mock' edition of *Australian Social Work*, the journal of the Australian Association of Social Workers. The theme for the special edition is 'Critical reflection: generating theory from practice'. Students are asked to use Fook's critical incident technique (Fook, 2002: 98–100) of deconstruction, reconstruction and theory generation to examine a critical incident from their field education (Pockett and Giles, 2008). Many of these incidents involve situations where professional boundaries were challenged and then expressed as binary positions based on taken-for-granted assumptions in their relationships with clients, agencies and their own worldviews about being a professional social worker.

In deconstructing and reconstructing an incident where a personal relationship became a professional one, Evans (2008) states,

It is often suggested that professional relationships in social work share many similarities with more intimate relationships, such as that of friendship ... this incident for me where the client and the friend became the same individual for me, forced me to ask myself the question, 'what differentiates professional client relationships from other relationships?'.

(Evans, 2008)

... even in my critical incident in which no interaction occurred ... there has still been a shift in the power between us – from a friendship where the power is equally distributed to this new, silent and unacknowledged relationship where the power in knowing and the capacity for action rests entirely with myself.

(Evans, 2008)

In analysing the discourse of her developed narrative of a critical incident in child protection, Tseris states:

Implicit in the narrative is the idea of equality between clients and practitioners, both of whom are seen as being free to express their views. I am surprised now as to how easily I had glossed over the agency context in which I was working. Little acknowledgement is made of the limitations and challenges of utilizing strengths-based approaches in child protection, and of the statutory power that is retained by social workers, regardless of the stage of intervention.

(Tseris, 2008: 36)

The sophistication and depth of these analyses demonstrates the final-year students' ability to both develop and critique a narrative using knowledge-creating approaches.

The final stage of the application of the model in the programme includes the articulation and labelling of students' new theories of practice. The capstone assignment provides a means through which students can confidently demonstrate the move from prescribed theoretical perspectives to the critical analysis of these perspectives based on their individual experiences in a practice context. Mastery over the curriculum content is enriched by confident critical inquiry that interrogates assumptions, values and power relationships. A teaching technique that supports this process is the use of 'critical friends', where students are paired up with a partner to critique individual experiences and responses to the critical incident. These approaches are supported by an educational culture in which the small group learning environment is respected, accepted and trusted by students and educators. The workshop approach used by the Fook and Gardner model is comparable to this small group learning environment, which is a cornerstone of the educational approach within the programme. Throughout the final two years, small group work provides a safe learning environment for experiential learning and the 'risk-taking' required in the critical task.

Sustaining new learning for change

The desired outcomes of the programme are consistent with those of most university-led professional degree programmes. The particular emphasis on critical reflection and transformational learning embeds concepts that support lifelong learning and confidence in critical inquiry, the development of new theories for practice, and the translation of these into change-related practice. Developing critically reflective social work graduates has, in our experience, proved to be an essential but complex developmental process. Long-term research has yet to be conducted to prove the efficacy of the processes we have developed. However, consistent feedback indicates that the graduates of this social work programme are highly respected for their critical thinking and action in practice. This deep learning leads to effective practitioners who can negotiate their way through the complexity of historical, structural and political factors; organisational, intrapersonal and interpersonal factors; considerations of theories for practice; considerations of codified values and ethics; and considerations of the exercise of power to the point of effective social transformation (Giles et al., 2010: 44). The integration into the programme of elements of the Fook and Gardner model and Fook's earlier approaches aids the achievement of these educational goals and supports students' learning, relationships with knowledge, and the transition to practice.

References

AASW (2010) *Australian Social Work Education and Accreditation Standards* (published March 2008, updated June 2009 and January 2010 to include addenda), Canberra, ACT: Australian Association of Social Workers.

Agger, B. (1998) *Critical Social Theories*, Boulder, CO and Oxford: Westview Press.

Barnett, R. (2007) *A Will to Learn*, Buckingham: Open University Press.

Biggs, J.B. (1978) 'Individual and group differences in study processes', *British Journal of Educational Psychology*, 48: 266–79.

——(1996) 'Enhancing teaching through constructive alignment', *Higher Education*, 32: 1–18.

Brookfield, S. (1995) *Becoming a Critically Reflective Teacher*, San Francisco: Jossey-Bass.

——(2009) 'The concept of critical reflection: promises and contradictions', *European Journal of Social Work*, 12(3): 293–304.

Clare, B. (2007) 'Promoting deep learning: a teaching, learning and assessment endeavor', *Social Work Education*, 26(5): 433–46.

Craddock, D., O'Halloran, C., Borthwick, A. and McPherson, K. (2006) 'Interprofessional education in health and social care: fashion or informed practice?', *Learning in Health and Social Care*, 5: 220–42.

Davidson, J. (2005) 'Professional relationship boundaries: a social work teaching module', *Social Work Education*, 24(5): 511–32.

Douglas, T. (2000) *Basic Groupwork*, London: Routledge.

Evans, M. (2008) 'When worlds collide: understanding the intersection of the personal and the professional in social work practice', in Pockett, R. and Giles, R. (eds),

Critical Reflection: Generating Theory from Practice. The Graduating Social Work Student Experience, Sydney: Darlington Press, 1–14.

Fook, J. (2002) *Social Work: Critical Theory and Practice*, London: Sage.

Fook, J. and Gardner, F. (2007) *Practising Critical Reflection: A Resource Handbook*, Maidenhead: McGraw Hill/Open University Press.

Giles, R., Irwin, J., Lunch, D. and Waugh, F. (2010) *In the Field: From Learning to Practice*, South Melbourne: Oxford University Press.

Irwin, J. and Napier, L. (2004) '(Re)forming field education: creating opportunities to maximise students' learning on placement', *Women in Welfare Education*, 7: 106–17.

McCune, V. and Entwistle, N. (2011) 'Cultivating the disposition to understand in 21st century university education', *Learning and Individual Differences*, 21: 303–10.

O'Hara, A. (2011) 'Introduction to working with groups', in O'Hara, A. and Pockett, R. (eds), *Skills for Human Service Practice: Working with Individuals, Groups and Communities*, South Melbourne: Oxford University Press, 226–53.

O'Hara, A. and Pockett, R. (2011) *Skills for Human Service Practice: Working with Individuals, Groups and Communities* (2nd edn), South Melbourne: Oxford University Press.

Payler, J., Meyer, E. and Humphris, D. (2007) 'Theorizing interprofessional pedagogic evaluation: framework for evaluating the impact of interprofessional continuing professional development on practice change', *Learning in Health and Social Care*, 6: 156–69.

Payne, M. (1982) *Working in Teams*, Basingstoke: Macmillan.

Pockett, R. and Giles, R. (2008) *Critical Reflection: Generating Theory from Practice. The Graduating Social Work Student Experience*, Sydney: Darlington Press.

Polanyi, M. (1967) *The Tacit Dimension*, New York: Doubleday.

Prosser, M., Trigwell, K., Hazel, E. and Gallagher, P. (1994) 'Students' experiences of teaching and learning at the topic level', *Research Development in Higher Education*, 16: 305–10.

Taylor, C. and White, S. (2000) *Practising Reflexivity in Health and Welfare: Making Knowledge*, Buckingham: Open University Press.

——(2006) 'Knowledge and reasoning in social work: educating for humane judgement', *British Journal of Social Work*, 36: 937–54.

Tseris, E. (2008) 'Examining these words we use: "participation", "empowerment" and the child protection role', in Pockett, R. and Giles, R. (eds), *Critical Reflection: Generating Theory from Practice. The Graduating Social Work Student Experience*, Sydney: Darlington Press, 30–44.

18 An online critical reflection dialogue group

Gail Baikie, Carolyn Campbell, Jackie Thornhill and Jodi Butler

Introduction

The Fook–Gardner model was re-theorized for alignment with our school of social work's critical philosophy and methodologically adapted for a web-based university course platform. The Critical Reflection Dialogue Group (CRDG) is now a core component of both the campus-based and distance delivery offerings of Bachelor of Social Work (BSW) program. Our discussion and analysis of the CRDG is organized into the following categories: Organizational culture and purpose; Theoretical orientation; Online CRDG pedagogical method; Preliminary analysis and insights. First, we ground this initiative within an institutional context that is historically situated and remains committed to enacting and teaching critical social work, as this accounts for the underlying theoretical emphasis and nuanced approach. The CRDG online version is then described with reference to recent literature on web-based forums for reflection and dialogue. In the end, we offer our initial insights from a research study in which we investigate the dialogical texts generated over the first two years. In the end, we acknowledge the magnitude of any undertaking that strives to contribute to the creation of critical social workers and muse about online forums as a possible means of further integrating critical reflection into the field, including the prospect of providing ongoing support to aspiring critical social work practitioners.

Organizational culture and purpose

The integration of a critical reflective orientation and the advent of the online CRDG mark an important chapter in our story as students, educators, professional social workers and CRDG facilitators within the School of Social Work at Dalhousie University in Halifax, Nova Scotia, Canada. Our critical philosophy has evolved since the 1970s, when the school had an explicit feminist identity and a 'radical social work' (Bailey and Brake, 1975) practice orientation. We have since embraced the contemporary tenets of structural (Mullaly, 2007), anti-racist (Dominelli, 1988), anti-oppressive (Dominelli, 1998), affirmative postmodernism (Leonard, 1994) and critical (Ife, 1997) social work orientations. Hence we have upheld a transformative framework for social work education and professional practice (Dominelli, 1998) and a vision of social work practice as a means to re-right unjust social relations (School of Social Work, 2011).

Critical thought and social work theory are now the foundation of our curriculum. Our critical culture, in addition to the action-oriented scholarship of past and present faculty, has led to strategies that bring together students and faculty with diverse individual and group identities, cultures and experiences. While these initiatives are integral to our agenda, they are insufficient, and we have also recognized that our responsibilities extend to constructing a 'critical culture of belonging' (Campbell and Baikie, 2012) beyond the classroom.

Despite these efforts, the student body continues to be disproportionately 'white' and mainstream. Even though students often become proficient with respect to the critical content, many will continue to use resistance strategies (Gay and Kirkland, 2003) when relating to other students and to faculty in a manner that challenges their dominant beliefs and assumptions of 'truth'. These strategies divert students who 'know better' from examining their privileged perspectives and resorting to their default assumptions (Lopes and Thomas, 2006). While capable of taking an 'observer stance' and critiquing overt and externalized instances of oppression, they are less likely to recognize the intangible and subtle ways in which they are complicit with domination and otherwise uphold and reproduce oppressive power relations through their everyday interactions. We are often perplexed that, despite our best efforts to enact our critical 'expertise', we continue to observe that our highly capable students resort to perceptions and interpretations of their subjective classroom and field experiences using pre-existing non-critical habits of mind (Mezirow, 1990) that are grounded in unrecognized and unquestioned assumptions, values and beliefs. This is disconcerting, given that their mindsets ultimately have more influence than substantive knowledge on the decisions practitioners make (Kumaş-Tan, 2005). This may be one reason why many critically trained social workers are observed to resort to mainstream perspectives and approaches when encountering the often 'hostile' (Greenman and Dieckmann, 2004) practice environment.

Our attempts at critically congruent organizational and pedagogical practices (Campbell, 2002) often engender strong emotive reactions that ignite tensions and conflict. Our response is guided by the view that the learning community is a microcosm of society. We are compelled to model engagement in a 'discourse of possibility' (McDonough, 2009) through strategies that evoke critical consciousness (Gay and Kirkland, 2003) and reconfigure intergroup interactions. Hence what is often perceived as 'a problem' actually provides an experience-based learning opportunity to acknowledge, scrutinize and reconfigure beliefs, ideas and practices that uphold domination and privilege. The Fook–Gardner critical reflection model offered us a strategic practice for facilitating the transition of these intersubjective events into teachable and transformative learning moments. The CRDG, which uses an adaptation of this model, provides one forum for this to occur. The CRDG is offered on-campus and online in order to maximize accessibility to both campus and distance BSW students (MSW students are invited, but we don't yet have a specific agenda for the MSW program). Participation in the CRDG is a mandatory component of one introductory course and is encouraged in several other courses. As a pedagogical tool, it supplements the critical content, reflective analysis and practice skills offered throughout the curriculum.

The CDRG forum reinforces critical reflection as a cornerstone of critical social work education and practice, and serves the following organizational (cultures of belonging) and pedagogical (consciousness-raising) and critical reflection skill development) goals:

- fostering respectful relationships through a genuine understanding of difference through a process of deconstructing the ways that dominant ideological, discursive, and structural influences are replicated in 'everyday' personal, professional, and institutional experiences and interactions
- facilitating the transformation to critical social work mindsets by surfacing and analysing the individual problematic cognitive meaning structures that prohibit genuine understanding of difference and the subsequent valuing of diversity
- supplementing critical course content with the development of the analytical skills and perspectives required for critical professional social work practice.

Theoretical orientation

While a vast repository of literature exists, most academic accounts describe a somewhat confusing array of critical reflection theorizations: some describe frameworks, strategies and practices, while only a few offer findings from research studies. While consistent with the Fook–Gardner model, our approach places more emphasis on socio-cultural theorizing. Transformational and experiential learning theories are core influences on the CRDG, but are extensively embellished with intercultural, critical, Freirian and feminist pedagogies.

Mezirow (1997) explains that transformational learning is 'the process of using a prior interpretation to construe a new or revised interpretation of the meaning of one's experience in order to guide future action' (p. 162). The focus of change is on the learners' 'frame of reference', which is composed of 'habits of mind' (ibid). Critical reflection is integral to transforming these cognitive meaning perspectives that have been established and entrenched through (exclusive or inclusive of Euro-Western) cultural assimilation (Mezirow, 1990). Mezirow's (1990) ideas stem from the notion of 'communicative learning', which entails a focus on 'understanding the meaning of what others communicate'; a recognition that these meanings are 'norm-governed'; and a 'critique of the relevant social norms and … cultural codes' that determine what is or is not acceptable (p. 8).

Mezirow's cognitive bent merges well with the liberation intent of Paulo Freire's model of co-intentional learning (Pietrykowski, 1996) and with the 'attitudinal transformations' (Nagda, 2006: 273) required for transcultural learning. Nagda (2006) points out that psychological, pedagogical and communicative pedagogical strategies are all necessary to ensure meaningful intergroup encounters. Popa and Cozma (2009) offer a helpful way to explain the integration of intercultural, critical and feminist pedagogies which underpin the CRDG. These orientations share the principle that education is a means to social change. Intercultural approaches emphasize the need to build relations through genuine dialogue and opportunities for collaboration. Critical pedagogy expands the thinking to other social group experiences, and promotes 'liberation by deconstructing the relation between power and culture' (p. 4), including those that are marginalized; emphasizing processes that enable dialogue, reflection and social critique, and promoting collective actions. Feminist approaches aim to build learning environments that are egalitarian, foster community, and value personal experience. Together these approaches also challenge the hegemonic notion that there is only one legitimate way to know the world, and related pedagogical practices strive to open space for multiple perspectives that stem from micro- and macro-collective worldviews.

Online CRDG pedagogical method

Our School is part of a more global trend that centers societal pluralism and online technology (Gaudelli, 2006) through offering our BSW and MSW programs online as well as on-campus. As a foundational component of the BSW curriculum, the CRDG was transitioned from its on-campus origins to the online platform. Recent scholarship in this area profile the use of online technology for uncovering cultural values and promoting cross-cultural interaction (Lin and Kinzer, 2003), exploring the doctrine associated with the development of intercultural understanding (MacPherson, 2010), providing professional peer support (DeWert et al., 2003), its use as a reflective evaluation tool (Glowacki-Dudka and Barnett, 2007), and its use as a platform for critical discussion and skill-building (Garrison et al., 2001; Watts and Lawson, 2009; Rocco, 2010). Still, 'little is known about the potential and means of the online setting as an avenue for transformational learning' (Taylor, 2007: 175).

Our CRDG forum may be the first web-based adaptation of the Fook–Gardner model (Fook, personal communication, 2010), and is at the leading edge of transformational online pedagogy. Oterholm (2009) used the Fook (2002) model as the basis for a learning exercise in a distance education course associated with social work field placements. However, the actual orientation to the model and modelling of the method were provided by the instructor during a face-to-face component of the course. Information was posted online, and students were given the option of meeting either virtually or in person, and were left to ask critically reflective questions of each other.

In contrast, our CRDG forum is exclusively online, with a strong emphasis on skilled facilitation by either a faculty member or a highly trained teaching assistant. Hence the CRDG is a stand-alone, web-based, purposeful pedagogical method, as opposed to a course activity. However, some of our early work was similar to Oterholm's approach. In comparison with our on-campus experiences, in certain respects the online environment is preferable, given that participants write and then post as opposed to verbalize their reflections. These postings become 'artifacts of ideas of the mind' (Taylor, 2007: 182) that, by being 'captured' in text, are more accessible to the participants and facilitators. As facilitators, we are better positioned to provide 'explicit guidance' (p. 187). We also suspect that the relative anonymity of web-based forums is more conducive to the formation of a climate of trust, openness and support required for transformative learning (Taylor, 2007). Furthermore, there are fewer impediments to the amount and frequency of any one student's active participation.

Mezirow (1997) explains that 'The educator functions as a facilitator and provocateur rather than an authority on subject matter' (p. 11). Our facilitation goal is to move students individually and collectively through a critical reflective analysis of the story in a manner that exposes problematic habits of mind; explores the subtleties of power; and enable insights into the interconnection between our personal and collective experiences and macro-discursive and structural conditions. In order to achieve these goals within our context, the Fook–Gardner (2007) model was adapted in order to

- suit the online structure
- simplify the process for beginning students
- enable relatively quick uptake, as students do not go through a 'training' process
- enable group learning and unlearning through a process that starts but does not stay with a specific individual experience (the initial story serves as a catalyst for others to relate to through either recalling similar experiences or imagining themselves within a similar event)
- ground the process within the principles of an Indigenous 'talking circle', thereby explicitly integrating another way of knowing and being
- facilitate the ability of students to link theory to everyday experiences as opposed to a professional capacity to link theory to practice
- model, but not teach, the skill of posing critically reflective questions, as this has proven to be an advanced skill.

The university's Blackboard Learning System (BLS) provides the course site platform for the CRDG. All BSW students, campus and distance, are enrolled in, and have access to, the group sessions. MSW students are invited and enrolled if requested. Upon entering, students see the Course Content page that contains links to the facilitators' biographies; an orientation slide presentation; group participation guidelines; the criteria for stories; and core critically reflective questions. On a side bar menu, students can access Announcements; Calendar; Mail; and Discussions. Each group session, taking place on the Main Discussion Board, begins on a Monday and ends the following Sunday. A separate Topic is created for each session, and there are eight to ten sessions over each of the fall and winter semesters.

Students are expected to contribute throughout the week for a total period of about an hour and a half, which is comprised of reading, contemplating and responding in a manner that builds on prior postings. The facilitator follows a standard framework, but remains attentive and responsive to both the substantive discussion and the transformational learning process. The framework consists of soliciting a personal story or critical incident – through an 'Announcement', students are invited to submit a personal experience using the 'Criteria for a critical incident (story)'. The story is emailed to the facilitator, who ensures it is suitable before making it the first posting for the session.

Criteria for a critical incident (story)

A critical incident is a personal or practice situation or experience in which you were actively involved and became acutely aware of issues of difference – racism, sexism, homophobia, heterosexism, ageism, classism. These are likely situations in which you experienced stress, intense emotion, discomfort or conflict. The event may be either negative or positive and may or may not involve your direct work with clients (perhaps colleagues, other agencies). The event may be large or small.

Critical incidents consist of:

- a description of a situation that led to the incident, including the background and context
- a concrete description of the incident, including a brief description of your initial reaction and those of other significant people, but refraining from incorporating analysis and explanation
- an explanation as to why the incident was significant to you.

(adapted from Montalvo, 1999; Kemppainen, 2000; Fook and Gardner, 2007)

Considerations:

- It's best not to choose an incident that happened recently as your emotions may be still too strong, making it difficult to reflect.
- It's also best not to choose an incident that may have legal or serious professional ethics issues.
- Be sure to protect the identities of the people involved.
- As usual, action may be taken if information is reported on current or potential harm to children or elders.

Seeking initial assumptions: through first asking the contributor, then encouraging other participants to identify their own assumptions associated with the story, and then asking all participants to consider the possible assumptions from additional perspectives. Postings should begin with 'I assume … '.

Identifying core themes: through analysng the assumptions. The facilitator identifies three to four core themes relevant for critical social work practice. Often these themes are revealed as binaries, or core unexamined 'truths'. About a third of the way through, the facilitator establishes separate discussion threads for each theme, and posts probing questions to guide participants in identifying the individual and societal assumptions, values and beliefs associated with each theme.

Making personal-is-political connections: through facilitating lines of inquiry that first expose and explore the power dynamics and complexities inherent within the themes and unearthed during the discussion, and then connect these insights to macro-cultural and societal discourses and structures.

Facilitating: through importing or creating strategies to keep the process on track, such as reminding participants of the purpose, guidelines and structure; and further enabling the group members to link their personal experiences and interpretations to cultural and societal experiences, perspectives and worldviews. For instance, 'The Mirror' was created because we observed that participants needed to return to and re-ground their insights within themselves. Participants are asked to hold up 'The Mirror' to their own postings throughout a session, and to identify what is revealed with respect to their own complicity or resistance to the problematic perspectives profiled during the session.

Moving towards action: through asking participants, in the closing thread, to identify and share a pertinent insight from the session and to consider how it might influence future choices and actions.

Consistent with the principles of a talking circle, the following guidelines frame the dialogue within the groups:

- Keep hearts and minds open – be supportive.
- Ensure everyone gets a chance to share.
- Do *not* focus on problem-solving, content, or evaluating the actions/inactions of the storyteller.
- Use the *story* as a window to explore how the *personal* is connected to the *political* (societal).
- Use the critical reflective questions posed by the facilitators to explore the layers of assumptions, values and beliefs that play out at the individual level but are connected to organizational and societal 'cultures' – continue to ask yourself *'but, why?'*

- Contribute your thoughts and insights (to the extent that is comfortable) – how you connect to the experiences in the story; your assumptions, values and beliefs; the connections you make to the underlying assumptions, values and beliefs in society.
- Do *not* provide advice, criticize, judge or debate – the focus is on 'I' not 'You'.
- Respect the privacy and confidentiality of the people in the stories and the participants in the group.

Preliminary analysis and insights

The online forum inadvertently provided us with a unique opportunity to research transformative learning within the CRDG. We are currently analysing the text generated from two years of online dialogue, and offer here some of our preliminary insights. Unlike the verbal CRDG campus-based discussion, the online written texts more explicitly expose and make accessible both the problematic habits of mind that beginning students often bring to their social work education, and the shifts that occur during communicative interaction within a session. The CRDG engages students in an examination of their everyday experiences in order to disrupt what would otherwise be considered 'natural' or 'normal'. This process exposes the subtleties that can easily be missed through traditional educational means. Within the online CRDG, students have considered the nuances of:

- practising as a critical social worker
- complexity of perceptions associated with social issues, social locations, and organizational and social 'cultures'
- complexities inherent within morality, ethics, social norms, through questioning what is right/wrong? good/bad? and, who decides?
- the enactment of oppression, domination and privilege in everyday institutional and individual practices
- our own intentional/unintentional complicity
- internal/external struggles
- micro-practices that are acts of resistance and contribute to social change
- helping and being a helper
- professional/client binary
- power and how it is enacted by users, providers, institutions
- user/worker responsibilities and accountabilities
- eurocentric dominance.

While we observe shifts in mind-sets in response to interventions by facilitators or other participants, several interrelated and prevalent discourses continue to be evident as 'habits-of-mind'.

- The privileging of an objectivist way of knowing and learning: students view 'real learning' as the cognitive acquisition of 'facts' that confer them with 'expertise'. They are often oblivious to their own contradictions. For instance, students will often say 'the client is the expert', while diminishing their own and other students' knowledge that stems from personal or group-based experiences that are embodied and emotive, or associated with a culture. Despite acquiring insight into the complexity and uncertainty of professional practice, they maintain expectations of being told the 'right' way to practice. Many have great difficulty being reflective and, when they are, will maintain the assumption that their interrelating is, and will be, unbiased and non-judgemental.
- A 'deficit' lens: service users are first, and often only, known through their 'problems', creating limited perceptions of weakness and vulnerability and assumptions of the need for expert help. The us/them binary is further solidified, precluding egalitarian, respectful and collaborative relations and the creation of alternatives.
- Individualism: given that the 'sanctity of the individual' is entrenched within Euro-Western society and the helping professions, students are primed to utilize individualist interpretations of social phenomena. They struggle first to comprehend their personal experiences as characteristic of social group experiences, and then make links to socio-political materialist and discursive contexts. The notions that 'individuals make and are responsible for their own choices'; 'difference is only a problem if you see it'; or 'equality means treating everyone the same' are prevalent and serve to maintain a 'blame the victim' ideology in which the 'victim' is sometimes the immoral and incompetent social worker.
- The dominance of biomedical and psychological understandings of human behaviour: given popular culture and their prior university courses, psychological, biomedical and psycho-social theories of human behaviour are typically the interpretive lens through which students determine 'truth'. Despite varying degrees of sociological, anthropological, political and educational theoretical knowledge (Campbell and Baikie, 2012), most have great difficulty interpreting micro-issues from these macro-frames.
- The 'othering lens': the dominant stance within both anti-oppression and diversity work entails the unproblematized assumption that a practitioner can become 'helpful' by coming to know 'the other' through learning about and from people who are marginalized or oppressed. Students frequently say this is the first time they are required to shift their gaze from the 'other' or the 'issue' to themselves and their own complicity. Having entered social work as moral people wanting to help others, many find it disconcerting that they themselves may be 'a problem', and may even question the validity of their education.

Given the hegemony of these fundamental assumptions, we do not blame students, and in fact would be surprised to find it otherwise. Not all students enter the program with, or maintain, these mindsets. Some, particularly those from marginalized identities, have had life experiences and other influences that configure their mindset differently, or at least have had previous cause to question the taken-for-granted 'norm'.

- While durability remains uncertain, the CRDG forum is extremely useful for exposing, and thereby enabling, the deconstruction and reconstruction of these perceptions. Also revealed are intriguing facets of the interaction between the 'self' and 'others'. For instance, students tend to assume another participant has a mainstream identity and 'normal' experiences unless they divulge their differences. Nevertheless, students do often come to sometimes quite profound insights and usually find the experience positive and practical, an achievement we relish, given that navigating the terrain of fundamental and sometimes sacred values and beliefs is inherently risky, and often avoided by both educators and students. During the 'Closing Circle' discussion thread, participants have: found the process 'enjoyable' and 'worthwhile'; 'unlearned' and feel 'enlightened' and 'enriched'; recognized the power inherent in asking or not asking critically reflective questions; a sense of 'personal growth' and 'healing'; grasped the 'invisibility of privilege' and the embedded nature of dominant discourses; comprehended the notion that social locations are not natural but socially constructed; questioned their own 'truths', including scared notions of themselves as being 'open', 'accepting' and 'non-judgemental'. Furthermore, students vow to continue to critically reflect, to remain vigilant, to avoid complacency, and to 'really listen' with 'humility'. These are encouraging indicators of an enhanced capacity to be critical social workers. Overall, participants appear to appreciate the opportunity to use course content to make sense of their individual and group-based experiences. Many also seem to appreciate our expectation for, and belief in, their abilities to think, analyse and contribute their knowledge meaningfully.

Conclusion

Within the CRDG space, we routinely experience both the exhilaration characteristic of a stimulating and thoughtful discussion, and the despair associated with the continuous resurfacing of mindsets that stem from Eurocentrism, capitalism and other oppressive ideologies. But we also observe, and many students self-report, that they are changed personally and professionally, as they no longer see society in quite the same way. The complacency associated with privilege is disturbed, and that which is ignored and dismissed, illuminated. Students now ask more penetrating questions and make more conscious and thoughtful decisions. Admittedly, we have overestimated our capacity as educators and as a school to incite complete transformation. Perhaps that is why we chose to identify ourselves as an 'aspiring' critical school of social work. Given these encouraging indications that many

students and graduates are also 'aspiring' critical social workers, we are somehow able to maintain our 'critical hope' (James et al., 2010: 27). The CRDG,
then, is not only a learning space, but also a platform for supporting and
promoting our individual and collective aspirations for critical social work
practices that withstands the contrary influences from within ourselves and
from within the field. Furthermore, the online medium opens up additional
possibilities for transitioning the essence of the CRDG to the field in forums
associated with field practicum supervision, professional development and
workplace supervision. Finally, the prospect of an ongoing online support
community for 'aspiring' critical social workers has begun to play in our
imaginations. While the challenges associated with transformational pedagogy remain, as teachers and learners we are encouraged by these possibilities, and remain motivated by so many of our students whose capacities
have blossomed within the context of our vigilance, scrutiny and critically
conscious and intentional teaching practices.

References

Bailey, R. and Brake, M. (1975) *Radical Social Work*, London: Edward Arnold.
Campbell, C. (2002) 'The search for congruency: developing strategies for anti-oppressive
social work pedagogy', *Canadian Social Work Review*, 19(1): 25–42.
Campbell, C. and Baikie, G. (2012) 'Beginning at the beginning: an exploration of
critical social work', *Critical Social Work*, 13(1): 67–81.
DeWert, M.H., Babinski, L.M. and Jones, B.D. (2003) 'Safe passages: providing
online support to beginning teachers', *Journal of Teacher Education*, 54(4): 311–20.
Dominelli, L. (1988) *Anti-Racist Social Work*, London: Macmillan.
——(1998) 'Anti-oppressive practice in context', in Adams, R., Dominelli, L. and
Payne, M. (eds), *Social Work: Themes, Issues and Critical Debates*, Houndmills:
Macmillan, 3–22.
Fook, J. (2002) *Social Work: Critical Theory and Practice*, London: Sage.
Fook, J. and Gardner, F. (2007) *Practising Critical Reflection: A Resource Handbook*,
Maidenhead: Open University Press.
Garrison, D.R., Anderson, T. and Archer, W. (2001) 'Critical thinking, cognitive
presence, and computer conferencing in distance education', *American Journal of
Distance Education*, 15(1): 7–23.
Gaudelli, W. (2006) 'Convergence of technology and diversity: experiences of two
beginning teachers in web-based distance learning for global/multicultural education',
Teacher Education Quarterly, 33(1): 97–116.
Gay, G. and Kirkland, K. (2003) 'Developing cultural critical consciousness and self-
reflection in pre-service teacher education', *Theory into Practice*, 42(3): 181–87.
Glowacki-Dudka, M. and Barnett, N. (2007) 'Connecting critical reflection and group
development in online adult education classrooms', *International Journal of Teaching
and Learning in Higher Education*, 19(1): 43–52.
Greenman, N.P. and Dieckmann, J.A. (2004) 'Considering criticality and culture as
pivotal in transformative teacher education', *Journal of Teacher Education*, 55(3):
240–55.
Ife, J. (1997) *Rethinking Social Work: Towards Critical Practice*, Melbourne: Longman.

James, C., Este, D., Bernard, W., Benjamin, A., Lloyd, B. and Turner, T. (2010) *Race and Well-being: The Lives, Hopes and Activism of African Canadians*, Halifax: Fernwood.

Kemppainen, J.K. (2000) 'The critical incident technique and nursing care quality research', *Journal of Advanced Nursing*, 32(5): 1264–71.

Kumaş-Tan, Z.O. (2005) 'Beyond cultural competence: taking difference into account in occupational therapy', Master's thesis, Dalhousie University, Halifax.

Leonard, P. (1994) 'Knowledge/power and postmodernism', *Canadian Social Work Review*, 11(1): 11–25.

Lin, X. and Kinzer, C.K. (2003) 'The importance of technology for making cultural values visible', *Theory into Practice*, 42(3): 235–42.

Lopes, T. and Thomas, B. (2006) *Dancing on Live Embers: Challenging Racism in Organizations*, Toronto, ON: Between the Lines.

MacPherson, S. (2010) 'Teachers' collaborative conversations about culture: negotiating decision making in intercultural teaching', *Journal of Teacher Education*, 61(3): 271–86.

McDonough, K. (2009) 'Pathways to critical consciousness: a first-year teacher's engagement with issues of race and equity', *Journal of Teacher Education*, 60(5): 528–37.

Mezirow, J. (1990) 'How critical reflection triggers transformative learning', in Mezirow, J. and Associates (eds), *Fostering Critical Reflection in Adulthood: A Guide to Transformative and Emancipatory Learning*, San Francisco: Jossey-Bass.

——(1997) 'Transformative learning: theory to practice', *New Directions for Adult and Continuing Education*, 74: 5–12.

Montalvo, F.F. (1999) 'The critical incident interview and ethnoracial identity', *Journal of Multicultural Social Work*, 7(3/4): 19–42.

Mullaly, B. (2007) *The New Structural Social Work* (3rd edn), Don Mills, ON: Oxford University Press.

Nagda, B.A. (2006) 'Breaking barriers, crossing borders, building bridges: communication processes in intergroup dialogues', *Journal of Social Issues*, 62(3): 553–76.

Oterholm, I. (2009) 'Online critical reflection in social work education', *European Journal of Social Work*, 12(3): 363–75.

Pietrykowski, B. (1996) 'Knowledge and power in adult education: beyond Freire and Habermas', *Adult Education Quarterly*, 46(2): 82–97.

Popa, N.-L. and Cozma, T. (2009) 'Crossroads on the way towards educational and social inclusion: intercultural, critical, and feminist pedagogy', *Acta Didactica Napocensia*, 2(1): 1–8.

Rocco, S. (2010) 'Making reflection public: using interactive online discussion board to enhance student learning', *Reflective Practice: International and Multidisciplinary Perspectives*, 11(3): 307–17.

School of Social Work (2011) 'Vision, Mission and Guiding Principles', School of Social Work, Dalhousie University, http://socialwork.dal.ca/Prospective%20Students/Vision%2C_Mission_and_.php

Taylor, E.W. (2007) 'An update of transformative learning theory: a critical review of the empirical research (1999–2005)', *International Journal of Lifelong Education*, 26(2): 173–91.

Watts, M. and Lawson, M. (2009) 'Using a meta-analysis activity to make critical reflection explicit in teacher education', *Teaching and Teacher Education*, 25: 609–16.

Conclusion

19 Implementing critical reflection in health and social care settings

Jan Fook

This book began with an outline of the contemporary issues facing the practice of critical reflection. These include the need to know and understand more about the varying ways it is practised; the need to know and understand more about the nature of the benefits that are accrued from its practice, particularly given the changing and challenging nature of workplace contexts; and the need for practical knowledge about how critical reflection might be adapted, and contribute, to the organisational context. So how is critical reflection practised in health and social care settings? What kinds of issues and difficulties arise, and what kinds of adaptations need to be made for specific uses and contexts? What do we learn about how critical reflection might be better practised and theorised? This chapter focuses on the themes that arise from the chapters in response to these questions. It is organised in the following way.

First, how the critical reflection model is actually used and modified is summarised, then specific benefits are outlined. Particular practical difficulties and other issues that arise from this are then discussed. The next two sections focus on specific contextual issues, and implications for learning at organisational levels. The final section discusses the implications for further theorising of critical reflection.

How was the critical reflection model actually used and/or modified?

Clearly – and this is hardly surprising – how the model was used depends to a large degree upon the purpose/s for which it was used, and I will discuss these differences shortly. In broad terms, though, it is clear that the model was either used almost identically to the 2007 outline, or was specifically modified for more particular usage. About half the chapters outline more specific modifications, and these tend to be the chapters focusing on teaching/ learning in particular programs outside the workplace (in formal degree programs in universities) or on research usages. Contributors who use the model in its more generic form tend to be more focused on supervision or learning in the workplace context. However, these tendencies are not hard and fast. The reasons for these different ways of using the model are many and varied. Delany and Watkin (chapter 16), who write about teaching in several different university programs, for instance, provide a nice way of understanding these different usages, ranging on a continuum from using the model in an identical way, to using more specific strategies to help students infuse the spirit of critical reflection. They also speak about needing flexibility in the way critical reflection is encouraged, in order to foster students' own responsibility for their own learning.

It is perhaps important to note that in situations where there are specific and stated learning goals, it may be more relevant to adapt the model to these purposes. For example, Baikie et al. (chapter 18) have developed the model very specifically for online use in a social work program based on critical principles. In this sense, too, their model emphasises the theoretical critical underpinnings, and focuses on helping students uncover assumptions that are relevant to this. They also point up the need to stage the expectations of what emerges from such a process at student level. They imply that a more fundamental learning from experience may be too advanced for students at this early stage.

Conversely, however, two other chapters (Lynne Allan's and Riki Savaya's) discuss using the more generic model in social work teaching: one in student supervision within field education, and one in a Master's degree programme. What is different about these usages is that the field education is located in the placement organisation (and therefore the learning focused on may be more generic) and the Master's programme deliberately sets out to teach reflection more generally. It does appear, broadly, that more generic approaches may be best suited to workplace situations where a range of both personal and organisational benefits may accrue (see for example Hickson's chapter 5). The range of benefits may also include team-building (see chapter 4 by Thomson), debriefing, support, or surfacing unpleasantness (see chapter 7 by Ferguson) or dealing with anxiety in the workplace (chapter 11 by Hearne), as well as more general learning from experience. This broad approach may also be more relevant in formal courses, where the aim is to teach people how to critically reflect as a set of skills, rather than focusing on predetermined specific learning goals. When it is used in a more precise fashion, it may be to help confront difficult assumptions and to clear barriers to palliative care referral (as in chapter 2, where McLoughlin and McGilloway use it in a workshop to assist palliative care health professionals); in raising critical awareness (as in chapter 18, where Baikie et al. use it to bolster the critical ideals of their social work program); or in enhancing other goals (such as in chapter 16, where Delany and Watkin discuss several different adaptations of the model for use in four different programmes with a range of other strategies, or in chapter 3, where Gardner illustrates how critical reflection can be integrated with spirituality to enhance a sense of critical spirituality). Interestingly, other literature notes the use of reflection to support other learning goals such as integrating research evidence into clinical decision-making (Vachon et al., 2010).

Implementing critical reflection 235

Research uses stand out as being the arena where many more specific modifications are needed. Not only do all aspects of the process need to be more explicable (in order to be implemented in a transparent fashion), but it also needs to be more open for ethical scrutiny. The three chapters in this section (chapters 12–14) detail a meticulous thinking through of these aspects. Morley (chapter 14) is closest to using the whole two-stage model, in that she is partly investigating whether the process can be used to reconstruct the thinking of sexual assault workers in more empowering ways. Janet Allen (chapter 13), by contrast, pares the model down using an autoethnographic approach to research her own practice of spirituality and the impact of her own assumptions on this. Askeland (chapter 12) introduces a focus group phase in order to develop the common knowledge of Ethiopian social workers.

What is clear is that the model and process are adaptable to a range of uses and settings, but what these are does need careful and thoughtful planning. This means it can also be used successfully within a suite of different strategies (see chapter 17 by Giles and Pockett). It can therefore be helpful to have a variety of usages and modifications, as long as there is clarity and transparency about the reasons for these.

Benefits and outcomes of using the model

The contributors note a vast list of perceived benefits and outcomes of practising critical reflection in their specific ways. These include, in the mental health field, an increased ability to deal with uncertainty, difference, collaboration and complexity (see chapter 6 by Gardner). These kinds of results are reported elsewhere (Chi, 2010). Others commented that the process contributed to the empowerment (see also Fook and Askeland, 2006) of participants, and their ability to be non-judgemental (see chapters 7 and 14). Lynne Allan notes the importance of using the critical reflection model for self-care (chapter 9). The ways in which critical reflection helps to deal with the emotional aspects of practice, increase self-awareness, and free up blind spots (see Savaya, chapter 15) also has clear implications for improved practice and finding new practice strategies (chapters 7 and 13). Obviously there is the related potential for new knowledge, especially contextual knowledge, to be created (chapter 12). On a team level, trust may be increased, and people from different professions may be helped to see their commonalities (Gardner and Taalman, chapter 8).

Most of these observations about outcomes, whilst heartening, do not necessarily provide any new insights about what we can expect from engaging in critical reflection. Rather, they perhaps confirm the diversity of benefits that accrue from engaging in critical reflection. The review and evaluative research undertaken in 2007 also indicate this broad range of benefits, which includes practical, rational, emotional and values-based changes (Fook and Gardner, 2007: 143). There is more recent research, however, that supports the benefits for teams (Richards et al., 2009). Other research in medicine indicates a growing interest in using critical reflection to teach professionalism (Goldie et al., 2007; Branch, 2010).

Practical difficulties

What were the purely practical difficulties that dogged authors in implementing critical reflection in their different settings? There were several resounding themes coming out here. First is the simple issue of attendance at critical reflection sessions. Several people noted the difficulties of ensuring consistent attendance in busy and pressurised workplaces (chapters 7, 8), or when sessions had to be held some time apart (chapter 12). There was a related difficulty of sustaining the group culture, especially when the success of critical reflection depends to a large extent on maintaining the appropriate group climate and trust. Continuity is also a particular problem when using the process for research. Lack of continuity can also erode the ability to engage all participants in the process (chapter 8). Jeffrey Baker (chapter 10) raises really pertinent reflections about the difficulties of learning in a reflective way in a pressurised climate – how technique may triumph over process and contribute to a negative climate.

Several questions arise from these practical difficulties. For instance, should membership of critical reflection groups be open or more targeted? (see chapters 7 and 8). Will more targeted group membership ensure better attendance and commitment to the process? Lastly, practical issues arise over how to involve managers in taking responsibility for ensuring that critical reflection happens in a systematic way in the workplace.

These practical issues indicate a need to develop strategies for maximising continuity. For example, can new group members be oriented in a way that sustains previous group culture? Can the initial orientation to critical reflection include establishing a group culture that takes into account lack of continuity, perhaps? Can a group culture be developed whereby groups are less dependent on continuity to work? For instance, spending time in group sessions to identify the factors that make the group work (other than continuity) could help. In this way, factors such as the group climate, and how trust is developed in each session, might become more important.

Helping to establish a broader organisational culture that values reflection may also assist in helping workers to prioritise attendance. For example, selling critical reflection as being about developing a culture that values self-care (see Lynne Allan's chapter), debriefing (perhaps couched as minimising/preventing error), and learning from experience as key contributions to improved outcomes to service users may also help. Enlisting the aid of managers in creating a supportive climate for critical reflection could involve anything from involving managers in the training, to developing systematic policies and practices.

Other issues

What other issues, of a less practical nature, have arisen from the authors' accounts? Several contributors raise the question of how to sustain the appropriate group climate and culture. Jeffrey Baker addresses this beautifully in his reflections (chapter 10) on his own experience of facilitating critical reflections as a team manager. This question also arises for other authors, and is linked with the issue of lack of continuity of attendance discussed above.

A further issue relates to vulnerability. Janet Allen (chapter 13) discusses this in relation to her own vulnerability, but it applies in more general terms. How is the potential vulnerability of participants managed in order to create a safe enough space for reflection? (see Lynne Allan's chapter 9). And people's own background cultures may differ regarding norms of what is seen as too personal or private to be discussed in more public or professional forums (Fook and Askeland, 2006).

Reflexivity issues arise in several ways. Baker (chapter 10) discusses how his position as manager put him in a paradoxical position of trying to create an ongoing space for his team to critically reflect on the effects of managerialism. This issue goes to some of the heart of the problem of how critical reflection can be effectively sustained in organisational contexts, especially when it may be managerialism itself that creates many of the personally experienced crises for workers.

Reflexivity plays a particularly significant role when using critical reflection as part of a research methodology. The three chapters (12–14) that look specifically at research note how the role of the researcher needs to be clearly thought through, particularly in terms of how the researcher influences the results (or not). For instance, how do the roles of group facilitator and researcher overlap (or not)? Who are the researchers in a critical reflection group? In chapter 12, Askeland deals with this issue by arguing that participants are co-researchers. Indeed, it is plausible to develop an approach to the use of critical reflection as a research methodology which includes the notion that all participants are researchers. This approach might even be relevant to establish a more open learning culture (see Fook, 2011). These issues point to the idea that it is crucial, with a research use of critical reflection, to think through relations between researcher and researched (see chapter 14 by Morley). The question of researcher bias – in terms of influencing interpretations of material, but also in terms of influencing the process of collecting material – is also important.

Contextual issues

What issues arise out of differences in the contexts in which people worked with this critical reflection model? First, the differences surrounding how the model is used with different professional groups is important. In chapter 2, McLoughlin and McGilloway needed to change the language of several of the key aspects in order to make the model more palatable to palliative care workers. Accordingly, they changed the term 'assumptions', and spoke more about common patient stories as opposed to 'critical incidents'.

Gardner (chapter 6) notices how mental health practitioners were very comfortable with the emotional aspects of critical reflection, perhaps more so than other professional groups she had worked with. Baker (chapter 10) also raises the question of how appropriate it might be to provide a lecture on the theoretical foundations of the critical reflection model when using it in a workplace setting and not an academic setting. This latter point is particularly an issue that I believe needs further development. It involves questions of how much explicit interpretive frameworks are needed to enhance people's reflective abilities given their particular context. Will people critically reflect better, envision and use more perspectives, if these are made more explicit in the critical reflection process? Do theories need to be named to be effective, or can critically reflective questions be asked in ways that utilise theoretical frameworks in a 'back-door' kind of way? Does this help minimise the potential threat of privileging theory, and therefore make the ideas more readily able to be integrated into personal experience?

These sorts of questions may have different answers for different professional groups as well, depending on the disciplinary background and ease with particular social science and educational concepts. Perhaps approaches to critical reflection based on concepts of spirituality or Eastern religions might be more easily appreciated by professionals from health backgrounds.

With questions of context and the different approaches needed, we must return to the question of why critical reflection is being used, and for what specific purposes. This appears to be the key issue, especially when we are dealing with a process that is potentially holistic and open-ended, from which a variety of benefits are forthcoming. The following themes emerge in relation to this:

- How the model is used (generic model or specific modification) will depend to some extent on whether it is used in a workplace or formal educational setting. Early indications appear to be that more generic uses are better suited to the workplace, although there are several notable exceptions to this trend in the book. For instance, more generic uses might include: supervision; team-building; learning how to critically reflect and/or learn from experience; encouraging empowerment; supporting self-care; or debriefing. More specific uses tend to include: unearthing assumptions to address blocks in practice; unearthing assumptions to support other learning; or research to identify particular knowledge or the foundations of practice. Some of the specific uses are listed in more detail below.
- The audience or target population will necessitate variations. For instance, the type of professionals (health or social care) being engaged; whether participants are students or practising professionals; and what stages of education the students are at.
- The model can be used in flexible ways, either as a 'stand-alone' process in order to simply assist people to learn how to reflect; in a modified version for more specific learning purposes; or in a modified version as part of suite of strategies to enable reflection.

- If the model is used for research purposes, much more specific design is called for, and attention needs to be paid in particular to reflexivity issues, ethical issues, and issues regarding the relationship between researcher and researched.

The specific purposes for which critical reflection was used include:

- to address blocks in practice
- to complement other kinds of learning (e.g. about spirituality and meaning)
- for supervision
- to help practitioners develop their theory of practice
- to research practice
- to develop knowledge relevant to practice
- to empower practitioners
- to enable work with uncertainty and changing contexts
- to understand the impact of assumptions on practice
- to assist in making workplace transitions
- to develop skills in critical reflection
- to develop critical consciousness
- to assist in integrating practices, theory and values.

Clearly, how each of these goals is realised in context may differ. What this list serves to highlight, though, is that the way critical reflection is used may need to be designed with particular goals in mind. This will also influence how the framework is 'sold' to participants. Some goals are framed in terms of more specific outcomes, some in terms of addressing perceived 'problems', and others in terms of the more amorphous practices (e.g. supervision) that we take for granted should happen in the workplace. It is useful to think through who the target audiences for critical reflection are, and therefore which purposes will speak best to that audience in their specific context.

Implications for organisations

What learning are we able to take away that has implications for organisational practices and learning? Interestingly, most contributors worked with critical reflection in a way that was not directly targeted at the organisation as a whole, although most contributors started with a mandate at some level of the organisation to practise critical reflection at least at team level. The focus still appears largely to have been more for individual/team levels of benefit. Having said this, clear organisational benefits emerged. For instance, Thomson (chapter 4) notes how a shared picture of professional practice was built up and used to suggest the need for change in the organisation. In mental health services, Gardner (chapter 6) notes how individual assumptions about management and the organisation were unearthed, as well as a sense of being able to have individual influence within an organisational context. I will return to these points in the final section.

Several chapters point up the ethical issues involved in practising or researching critical reflection, especially when used for research purposes. How can individual safety be protected in work environments that may seek to blame individual performances? Some contributors emphasised the need to create safe places within these broader contexts. Perhaps having greater manager involvement in critical reflection might assist with this issue.

In some cases, although the critical reflection undertaken with specific groups was deemed successful, there did not appear to be a translation of this learning into other organisational forums (Gardner and Taalman, chapter 8). This apparent blockage is relevant to one of the key issues identified in the literature, which is about how individual learning becomes translated into organisational learning (Nonaka and Takeuichi, 1995; Crossnan and Lane, 1999).

Linking individual and organisational levels of learning is a key problem identified in the literature on organisational learning. For example, Perkins and Best (2007) conclude that organisations which empower individual learning are better able to learn organisationally, but that (interestingly) the learning should include features of what some of our chapters have identified happens in a critically reflective process (e.g. a focus on organisational values, power relationships, interdependence with the community, and working together for organisational change).

Further theorisation

Where does all this leave us in terms of our further understanding of critical reflection in context?

My reflections on re-reading all the chapters have led me to make a clearer delineation of both the different purposes for which critical reflection may be used, and the different ways it may be theorised. The uses of critical reflection range from using it as a tool to enhance other learning, to learning how to critically reflect (or learn from experience) in its own right. This latter type of use underscores the importance of experience as the raw material for learning (see chapters 8 and 12), so how experience (and learning) is understood and theorised is therefore crucial to the focus taken. Several chapters emphasise the emotional aspects of experience and learning (Hearne), but other chapters on spirituality tend to emphasise the meaning aspect.

The different theoretical perspectives we take does, on some level, boil down, for me, into a relatively simple dichotomy of whether we focus on the 'critical' or the 'reflection' aspect. Critical aspects focus on both the fundamentality of the reflection (and therefore the degree to which it is transformative), and the ability to raise one's critical awareness. The reflection aspects focus more on the ability to learn from experience. These are, of course, not mutually exclusive. However, critical social science theories have tended to inform the former, and the latter perhaps have been informed by adult learning theories, and now are also tending to be further informed by perspectives that emphasise the spiritual aspects of being. The latter theories focus more on meaning, and a holistic meaning as well – they focus on how interpretations are made of experience in a particular context, and how this can help develop broader principles for living that are transferable across contexts. Whist I am aware that this dichotomy can be seen as a gross oversimplification, I am also aware that it may be helpful to polarise the two sets of thinking in order to point up what I believe is now the task at hand – to theorise critical reflection in a more integrated way to allow for all aspects of experience to be included in a way that allows for a holistic and transformative approach to practise in context. Looking at the problem from this point of view means that attempts to theorise particular aspects of critical reflection (such as the emotions) do not really grapple with the bigger problem of how to enable a framework that allows personal experience and its meaning to be seamlessly integrated with a sense of power in context. This remains a challenge that is yet to be fully engaged with.

This type of need is evident in some of the organisational learning literature, which notes that learning is more than just learning new knowledge, but is also about how to 'be' and to 'do' in organisational context (Elkjaer, 2003). This has relevance when applied to critical reflection in organisations. In other words, what can be guided in critical reflection is a learning about identity, how to practise, and the relevant knowledge about this. This would accord with an approach to organisational learning that is about how individuals make sense of their organisations (e.g. Weick, 1995) and their place within them. This is supported by Argyris and Schön's (1996) thinking that organisational learning can be likened to learning about the political conditions under which individuals function as agents of organisational action. This way of putting it potentially conceptualises a link between individual and organisational learning and individual practice, and includes a power dimension.

A key way of thinking about critical reflection in an organisational context can therefore be to think about how critical reflection can directly link individual and organisational learning and practice, and in particular the political dimensions of this. To spell this out, critical reflection on individual workers' experiences can feed into organisational learning by helping to surface, examine and change the fundamental individual (and shared) assumptions about their organisations and their sense of identity ('being') within these. This, in turn, sparks new knowledge ('knowing') and a sense of how to change practice ('doing'). The latter represents the theory of practice (the goal of stage 2 critical reflections in our model), and is potentially transformative in that it enables a new way of enacting new or reaffirmed knowledge. In this way, people's sense of themselves, and their own power or sense of agency, can be integrated with new knowledge and new ideas of how to practise effectively in organisational contexts.

References

Argyris, C. and Schön, D. (1996) *Organisational Learning II: Theory, Method and Practice*, Reading, MA: Addison-Wesley.

Branch, W. (2010) 'The road to professionalism: reflective practice and reflective learning', *Patient Education and Counselling*, 80(3): 327–32.

Chi, F.M. (2010) 'Reflection and teaching as inquiry: examples from Taiwanese in service teachers', *Reflective Practice*, 11(2): 171–83.

Crossnan, M.M. and Lane, H.W. (1999) 'An organisational learning framework', *Academy of Management Review*, 24(3): 522–37.

Elkjaer, B. (2003) 'Social learning theory: learning as participation in social processes' in Eaterby-Smith, M. and Lyyles, M. (eds) *The Blackwell Handbook of Organisational Learning and Knowledge Management*, MA: Blackwell, pp. 38–53.

Fook, J. (2011) 'Developing critical reflection as a research method' in Higgs, J., Titchen, A., Horsfall, D. and Bridges, D. (eds) *Creative Spaces for Qualitative Researching*, Rotterdam: Sense Publishers, pp. 55–64.

Fook, J. and Askeland, G.A. (2006) 'The "critical" in critical reflection', in White, S., Fook, J. and Gardner, F. (eds), *Critical Reflection in Health and Social Care*, Maidenhead: Open University Press, 40–54.

Fook, J. and Gardner, F. (2007) *Practising Critical Reflection: A Resource Handbook*, Maidenhead: Open University Press.

Goldie, J., Dowie, A., Cotton, P. and Morrison, J. (2007) 'Teaching professionalism in the early years of a medical curriculum: a qualitative study', *Medical Education*, 41(6): 610–17.

Nonaka, I. and Takeuichi, H. (1995) *The Knowledge Creating Company*, New York: Oxford University Press.

Perkins, D. and Best, K. (2007) 'Community organizational learning', *Journal of Community Psychology*, 35(3): 303–28.

Richards, P., Mascarenhas, D. and Collins, D. (2009) 'Realizing reflective practice approaches with elite team athletes: parameters of success', *Reflective Practice*, 10(3): 353–63.

Vachon, B., Durand, M.J. and LeBlanc, J. (2010) 'Using reflective learning to improve the impact of continuing education in the context of work rehabilitation', *Advances in Health Sciences Education*, 15(3): 329–48.

Weick, K. (1995) *Sensemaking in Organisations*, London: Sage.

Index

Notes are indicated by suffix "n" (e.g. "164n3" means note 3 on page 164); "critical reflection" is abbreviated [in this index] as "CR", and "Fook–Gardner model" as "F/G model"

114, 115, 117, 118, 119, 127, 128, 130, 131, 132, 144, 145, 147, 154, 156, 166, 167, 169, 170, 171, 174, 175, 183, 184, 186, 187, 188, 196, 198, 202, 205, 208, 209, 210, 211, 213, 223, 224, 235
Garrick, J. 101
Garrison, D.R. 222
Gaudelli, W. 222
Gay, G. 220
Giles, R. 210, 213, 215, 217
Gilligan, P. 29, 31
Giroux, H. 166, 169, 170
Glowacki-Dudka, M. 222
Goldie, J. 236
Goleman, D. 62
Goodman, J. 170
Gould, N. 5, 61, 128
Grant, L. 61
Gray, M. 29, 31, 61
Greenman, N.P. 220
Gross, R.M. 30
group care: staff teams working in 87–8
groups: value of working in 39, 112
Gustafsson, G. 31

Hansen, E. 200
al-Haqq Kugle, S.S. 30
Hawkins, L. 33
Hawkins, P. 94, 106
Haynes, A. 28
Healy, K. 111, 145
Hearne, B. 127
Heelas, P.A. 30
Helmeke, K.B. 29
Hick, S.F. 77
Hickson, H. 58
Higgs, J. 170, 202, 206
Hodge, D. 30
Hoffman, L. 29
holistic ways of working 31, 40, 41
Holloway, M.A. 30
Howe, D. 89, 90
Hoyrup, S. 2
Huffington, C. 73, 102
Humphrey, C. 4
Humphreys, M. 155
Humphries, B. 169, 170, 171, 172, 173
Hunt, B. 29
Hunt, C. 4, 182

iceberg metaphor 72, 73, 76
Ife, J. 219
'impostor syndrome' 124

interdisciplinary team [in Australian health service] 93; CR used by 95–9; influence of CR on practice 99–101
intuitive skills 92
Ireland: palliative care 15–27
Irwin, J. 46, 208
Israel: Tel Aviv University MSW program 181–94
Ixer, G. 120

Jack, G. 85, 86, 87, 91
Jackson, M. 89
James, C. 229
Jankowicz, D. 21
Jensen-Hart, S. 155
Johns, C. 4, 31, 65, 200
Jones, C. 120, 121, 123, 125
Jones, S.H. 155
journal writing 60
judgemental questions: reaction to 121

Kadushin, A. 71, 94
Kamitsuka, M.D. 30
Kavanagh, J. 29
Kellehear, A. 7, 16, 17, 18, 27
Kelly, G.A. 15, 21
Kemppainen, J.K. 224
Kinman, G. 61
Kinzer, C.K. 222
Kirkland, K. 220
Kirkpatrick, M.K 17
'knowing in action' 154
knowledge concepts 3, 161–2
knowledge-creation principles 145
Knowles, M. 197
Knowles, M.S. 199, 201, 202
Kolb, D.A. 3
Kugle, Scott see al-Haqq Kugle, S.S.
Kumaş-Tan, Z.O. 220

La Trobe University [Australia] Centre for Professional Development: spirituality/CR workshops 32–7; supervision and CR training 94
Laabs, C. 31
Landfield, A.W. 24
Lane, H.W. 240
Lartey, E.Y. 30
Lave, J. 203, 204
Lawson, H. 87, 88
Lawson, M. 222
learning [about] CR 59–62; challenges encountered 62, 109–10
learning climate/culture 7–8

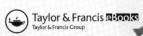